AF477881

Excimer
Laser Surgery
for Corneal Disorders

Excimer Laser Surgery for Corneal Disorders

Peter S. Hersh, M.D.

Director, Cornea and Refractive Surgery
Associate Professor of Ophthalmology
UMDNJ—New Jersey Medical School
Newark, New Jersey
Director, Cornea and Laser Vision Institute
Hackensack University Medical Center
Hackensack, New Jersey

Michael D. Wagoner, M.D.

Medical Director
Chair, Department of Ophthalmology
King Khaled Eye Specialist Hospital
Riyadh, Kingdom of Saudi Arabia
Cornea Service
Massachusetts Eye and Ear Infirmary
Department of Ophthalmology
Harvard Medical School
Boston, Massachusetts

1998

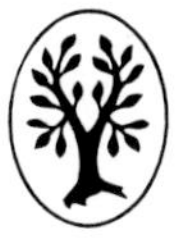

Thieme
New York • Stuttgart

Thieme New York, Inc.
333 Seventh Ave.
New York, N.Y. 10001

Excimer Laser Surgery for Corneal Disorders
Peter S. Hersh
Michael D. Wagoner

Library of Congress Cataloging-in-Publication Data

Hersh, Peter S.
    Excimer laser surgery for corneal disorders / by Peter S. Hersh
  and Michael D. Wagoner.
        p.   cm.
    Includes bibliographical references and index.
    ISBN 0-86577-686-5 (TMP). — ISBN 3-13-107961-4 (GTV)
    1. Cornea—Laser surgery.   2. Excimer lasers.   I. Wagoner,
  Michael D.
    [DNLM: 1. Corneal Diseases—surgery.   2. Keratectomy,
  Photorefractive, Excimer Laser.   WW 220H572e   1997]
  RE86.H47   1997
  617.7'19059—dc21
  DNLM/DLC
  for Library of Congress   97-18429
                                                                         CIP

Important note: Medical knowledge is ever-changing. As new research and clinical experience
broaden our knowledge, changes in treatment and drug therapy may be required. The authors
and editors of the material herein have consulted sources believed to be reliable in their efforts
to provide information that is complete and in accord with the standards accepted at the time
of publication. However, in view of the possibility of human error by the authors, editors, or
publisher of the work herein, or changes in medical knowledge, neither the authors, editors,
publisher, nor any other party who has been involved in the preparation of this work, warrants
that the information contained herein is in every respect accurate or complete, and they are not
responsible for any errors or omissions or for the results obtained from use of such information.
Readers are encouraged to confirm the information contained herein with other sources. For
example, readers are advised to check the product information sheet included in the package
of each drug they plan to administer to be certain that the information contained in this publication is accurate and that changes have not been made in the recommended dose or in the
contraindications for administration. This recommendation is of particular importance in con-
nection with new or infrequently used drugs.

Some of the product names, patents, and registered designs referred to in this book are in fact
registered trademarks or proprietary names even though specific reference to this fact is not
always made in the text. Therefore, the appearance of a name without designation as proprietary
is not to be construed as a representation by the publisher that it is in the public domain.

Printed in the United States of America

5 4 3 2 1

TNY ISBN 0-86577-686-5
GTV ISBN 3-13-107961-4

*This book is dedicated to my
mother, Carol A. Hersh*
—PH

To my family
—MDW

Contents

Preface ix

1. Introduction to Excimer Laser Technology 1

2. Case Selection and Surgical Decision Making 11

3. Techniques of Excimer Laser Phototherapeutic Keratectomy 36

4. Clinical Results 75

5. Complications 89

6. Refractive and Topographic Complications and Considerations 105

7. Phototherapeutic Keratectomy for Complications of Excimer Laser Refractive Surgery 129

Addendum: Case Studies 154

Index 157

Preface

The development of novel surgical techniques and adjunctive technologies continues to improve the treatment of patients suffering from corneal disorders. The lamellar structure of the cornea makes it uniquely suitable to conventional superficial surgery for a variety of superficial scars, dystrophies, and degenerations. In many cases, however, manual keratectomy leaves an irregular surface and residual scarring and opacity. Thus, the recent introduction of the excimer laser promises to give the corneal surgeon a unique tool to aid in superficial corneal surgery. Excimer laser-assisted keratectomy may clear superficial corneal opacities and leave a smooth, optically functional surface. In fact, some patients who heretofore required corneal transplantation may be helped by excimer laser-assisted superficial corneal surgery, more commonly referred to today as phototherapeutic keratectomy (PTK).

This book is structured to give the reader a resource detailing all aspects of the PTK procedure. Although based on the authors' experience and perspective, it draws heavily upon and reviews the growing body of literature available on the subject today. The first chapter presents an overview of the basic physics and laser tissue interaction underlying the photoablation process. Since the excimer laser operates on principles different from our typical surgical instruments, such background is necessary to understand and anticipate the tissue effects which will occur when treating patients.

Proper case selection is of paramount importance to insure a successful surgical outcome. Chapter 2, therefore, reviews the essentials of appropriate case selection and strategic surgical planning. Chapter 3 describes in detail those specific surgical strategies available. This chapter should guide the surgeon through the intricacies of the laser techniques which now are available to treat a wide variety of corneal disorders. Its goal is to walk the reader through the specific procedures, giving the surgeon a detailed blueprint of the selected technique. Each procedure is illustrated by clear line drawings and illustrative case studies.

Chapter 4 reviews the results of published studies to date. This should provide the reader with the information necessary to properly inform patients regarding the prognosis in their specific situation. In Chapters 5 and 6, we review the potential side effects of treatment and stress those strategies which can be employed to avoid complications of the PTK procedures. Finally, Chapter 7 discusses techniques of PTK which may be used to treat a number of complications resulting from excimer laser photorefractive keratectomy.

Throughout the book, specific case studies are used to illustrate the subject matter more clearly. Since PTK may be used to treat a number of different corneal disorders, and since surgical strategies are designed specifically for each case situation, excimer laser-assisted superficial corneal surgery is, in many cases, an art. Minor variations in technique may make the difference between a successful and unsuccessful result. Thus, clinical experience is vital to best treat the patient and a review of actual cases useful in becoming proficient with patient selection and the techniques of PTK. While case studies are presented throughout the text, they also are referenced conveniently in the Addendum.

We hope this book will be of use to the corneal surgeon, the general ophthalmologist, and the ophthalmologist-in-training. We also hope that *Excimer Laser Surgery for Corneal Disorders* will play a part in expanding our knowledge, expertise, and interest in this burgeoning field of corneal surgery.

We would like to gratefully acknowledge Laurel C. Lhowe of Cambridge, Massachusetts for again producing outstanding ophthalmology illustrations, and Andrea Seils of Thieme for her energetic efforts in bringing this project to fruition. Our thanks also to Rashna Irani of Boston University and Kevin Scher of Princeton University for their assistance in preparation of the manuscript.

Peter S. Hersh
Michael D. Wagoner

Excimer
Laser Surgery
for Corneal Disorders

◆ 1 ◆

Introduction to Excimer Laser Technology

Over the past decades, a variety of novel surgical techniques have evolved to treat many corneal disorders. These include advancements in penetrating and lamellar keratoplasty, superficial keratectomy procedures, and ocular surface surgery. Most recently, the excimer laser has emerged from the laboratory as a clinical surgical tool.[1-4]

Laser-assisted superficial keratectomy, commonly known as *phototherapeutic keratectomy* (PTK), has been a valuable corneal surgical modality for a number of years in the international community. In the United States, the use of the excimer laser for treatment of corneal surface diseases was approved by the U.S. Food and Drug Administration (FDA) in 1995. Unlike photorefractive keratectomy (PRK) for the correction of myopia, which gives the ophthalmologist a novel and unique total methodology for refractive surgery, the excimer laser, when used for superficial corneal surgery, simply provides a new tool in the traditional armamentarium of the corneal surgeon.

Whether PTK is used alone or as an adjunctive strategy in traditional mechanical superficial keratectomy techniques, a number of disorders affecting the corneal surface may be successfully treated because of the excimer laser's ability to meticulously remove superficial corneal tissue. Such disorders include a variety of corneal degenerations and dystrophies, corneal irregularities, and superficial scars. Clinical results have shown PTK to be helpful to patients suffering from superficial corneal opacities, scars, and irregularities.[5-9]

While some of these conditions heretofore could be treated satisfactorily by mechanical superficial keratectomy,[10,11] laser-assisted superficial keratectomy may minimize tissue removal and surgical trauma in some cases. The

"

therapeutic success of PTK relies both on the ability of the laser to meticulously remove tissue from the corneal surface and on the cornea subsequently to remain smooth, without scarring, and with adequate epithelial regeneration and adherence to the new corneal surface.[12–17] The smoother stromal surface that results from the photoablation process may improve surface optical topography, improve postoperative corneal clarity, decrease postoperative scarring, and facilitate subsequent epithelial adhesion. Moreover, some corneal disorders that would otherwise require lamellar or penetrating keratoplasty may be amenable to treatment with the excimer laser, obviating the need for more invasive surgery.

Surgical strategies will vary significantly with different corneal disorders, and the clinical goals of the PTK procedure, likewise, may vary depending on the patient's symptomatology. In addition, the side effects and complications of PTK may differ from those of both PRK and mechanical superficial keratectomy. Thus, the surgeon must practice careful case selection, devise an appropriate surgical strategy tailored to the individual patient problem, and properly execute the procedure to optimize clinical outcomes.

Given these considerations, the goal of this text is to review, in depth, indications and patient selection, surgical techniques, postoperative care, and complications of superficial corneal surgery using the excimer laser.

Excimer Laser Principles

The excimer laser is based on the combination of two gases—a noble gas and a halogen. Both of these are generally stable in their normal low energy state. When a high voltage electrical discharge is delivered into the laser cavity containing these gases, they combine to form a higher energy state compound. The term *excimer,* indeed, derives its name from a contraction of "*exc*ited *dimer.*" Upon the dissociation of this high energy compound, a photon of energy is released corresponding to the bond energy of the noble gas–halogen molecule.[18,19] This wavelength of light energy is amplified in the laser system, resulting in the production of a discrete, short duration, high energy pulse of laser energy (Fig. 1–1).

The specific wavelength of an excimer laser depends on the gases utilized. Excimer lasers in current clinical use rely on argon and fluorine gas to emit a wavelength of 193 nm, thus falling in the ultraviolet C range of the light spectrum. Although other gas mixtures will yield other laser wavelengths (for instance, the krypton fluoride excimer laser used in early laboratory studies emits at 248 nm),[20,21] 193 nm has been found to be the wavelength of choice for clinical procedures. Laser energy at 193 nm is very well absorbed by the proteins, glycosaminoglycans, and nucleic acids comprising the cornea. Since a 193 nm photon is of higher energy than the molecular bond strength of these compounds, absorption of the laser energy results in breaking of the bonds. Those molecular fragments that result are ejected from

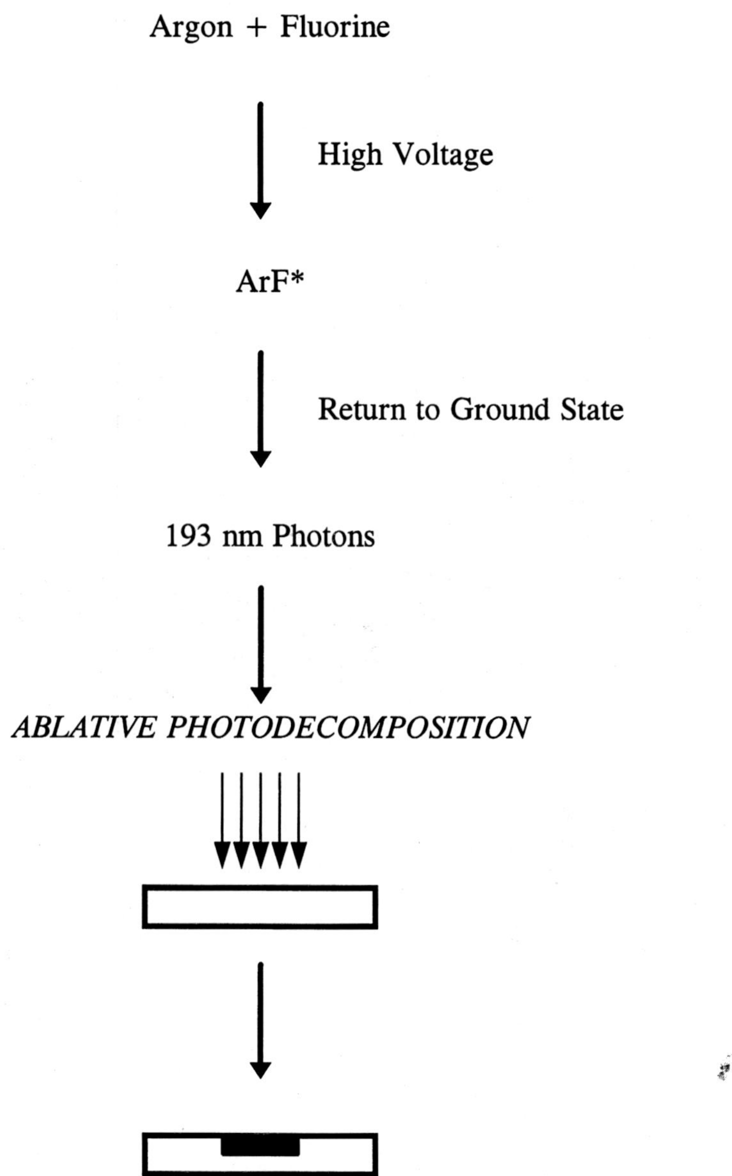

Figure 1–1.   Scheme depicting the release of a high energy photon of 193 nm emitted by the argon fluoride excimer laser and the photoablation process.

the surface of the cornea at supersonic speeds.[22,23] The excimer laser tissue removal process is termed *ablative photodecomposition.*[3] It is important to understand that the excimer laser does not cut tissue like a scalpel; rather, it ablates or removes tissue from the corneal surface. When used clinically, the ablated material appears as an effluent plume (Fig. 1–2). Analysis of this plume has shown it to consist of a variety of high molecular weight hydrocarbons.[24]

Excimer laser photoablation of corneal tissue takes place when the energy density per pulse (fluence) exceeds 50 mJ/cm^2.[25] Current excimer lasers in

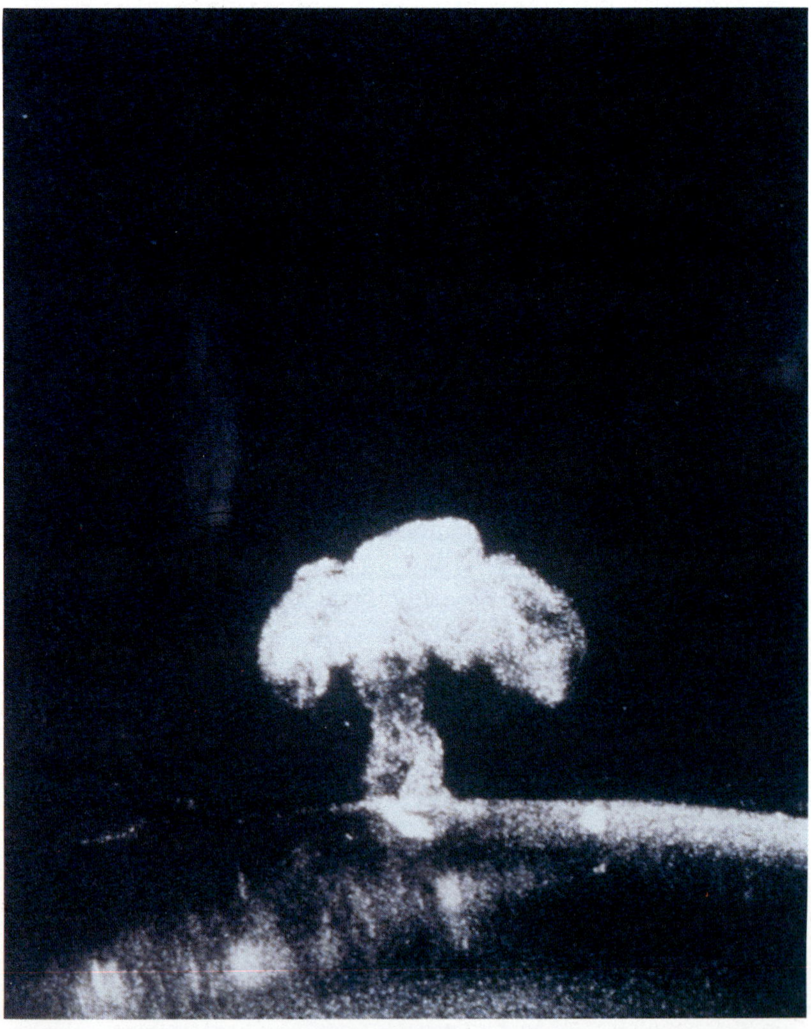

Figure 1–2. High speed photography showing excimer laser ablation effluent plume. (Reproduced with permission from Puliafito et al.[31] Copyright 1987, American Medical Association.)

clinical use operate at energy levels ranging from approximately 120 to 250 mJ/cm², pulse repetition rates of 5–20 Hertz, and a pulse duration of approximately 10–20 ns. The expected ablation rate of corneal tissue averages approximately 0.25 µm per pulse for an excimer laser operating at a fluence of 180 mJ/cm².[26–28] The ablation rate per pulse is somewhat lower for lasers operating at a fluence of 150 mJ/cm². Unlike PRK, which relies on computer-controlled delivery of the laser energy, the beam diameter in PTK is fixed while the energy and pattern applied are determined by the surgeon.

Laser Delivery

The excimer laser is comprised of the following components: (1) gases, (2) power source, (3) laser cavity, (4) beam-forming optics, (5) delivery system, (6) aiming system, and (7) surgical microscope. For most current excimer laser systems, the initial pulse delivered from the laser cavity is a broad rectangular beam of irregular energy level. For clinical use, this beam needs to be homogenized to yield a consistent energy over the entire delivery area. In the absence of a smooth and consistent beam energy, ablation rates could vary over the treatment zone, resulting in irregular tissue removal. In addition, the beam needs to be masked in two dimensions to the appropriate size and shape. Such beam homogenization and shaping are accomplished through a number of beam-shaping optics in the optical train of the laser. Moreover, a diaphragm[29] interposed within this optical train masks the beam, causing it to be delivered as a circular spot of a chosen fixed diameter (Fig. 1–3).

The energy and homogeneity of the laser beam must be verified before patient treatments. Preoperative laser calibration is necessary to ensure that the laser beam aiming system is aligned, that the cross-sectional beam homogeneity is acceptable, and that the ablation rate per pulse of the laser is

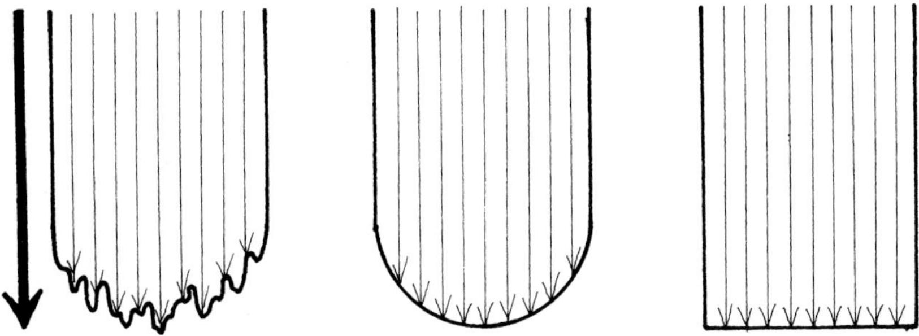

Figure 1–3. Excimer laser cross-sectional energy profiles. **(Left)** Irregular cross-sectional energy profiles. **(Center)** Gaussian energy distribution. Fluence is higher centrally than peripherally. **(Right)** "Flat-top" beam profile. Fluence is consistent across face of the entire laser beam.

within accepted tolerances. The different manufacturers of the lasers provide detailed procedures for assessing laser calibration. If laser performance does not conform to their guidelines, surgery is postponed and the laser is adjusted.

There are three general methods for ascertaining the energy output and homogeneity of the radiant energy density (beam profile) of the excimer laser. Most lasers currently available have an internal energy meter that indicates the energy of the laser during the treatment immediately preceding. Another method is to ablate materials of known thickness and ablation rate to provide a qualitative and semiquantitative analysis of the laser beam profile. Finally, several laser manufacturers use polymethylmethacrylate (PMMA) discs to monitor the ablation characteristics of the excimer laser in both a qualitative and quantitative manner (Fig. 1–4). Two types of measurement can be performed. The contour of the laser beam profile can be inferred from the PMMA ablation profile as measured by a scanning profilometer, which measures the sagittal depth of material removed, after ablation with a fixed beam diameter and a fixed number of pulses. For refractive procedures, in addition, the refractive accuracy of the laser on a given day can be checked. This involves the programming of the laser to perform a specified amount of PRK treatment. With some laser systems, the PMMA disc can be examined with a lensometer to measure the dioptric ablation achieved, and with others the disc is scanned with a profilometer to determine the sagittal depth of the ablation in all dimensions. Newer

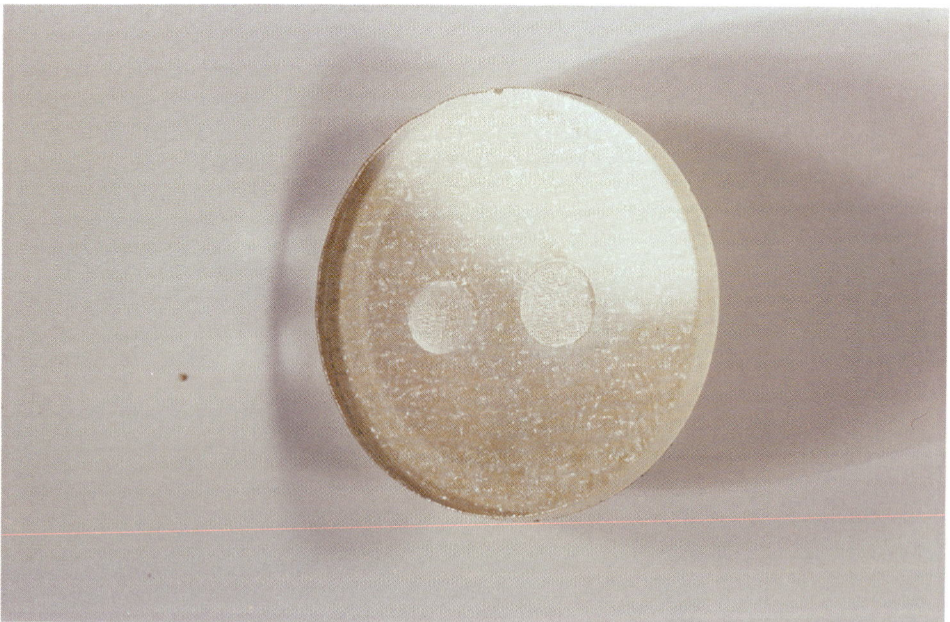

Figure 1–4.   Test ablations in a polymethylmethacrylate disc.

methodologies to more accurately measure the beam profile and ablation rate are currently under development.[30]

Laser–Tissue Interaction

There are a number of attributes of the argon fluoride excimer laser ablation that make it particularly appropriate for superficial corneal surgery. The laser energy is very well absorbed near the corneal surface and thus, theoretically, should have few deep direct or secondary acoustic shockwave effects on the corneal tissue. The ablation process is rapid, and excess energy is ejected with the effluent plume[31]; thus, there appears to be minimal thermal damage to the tissue as well.

Furthermore, unlike other lasers in use in ophthalmology, the excimer laser pulse is delivered as a relatively broad beam. Current lasers have beam diameters up to 6.5 mm. Over the entire area upon which the laser beam impinges, molecular bonds will be broken and tissue removed (Fig. 1–5). Hence, relatively large areas of the cornea can be treated with each pulse. Alternatively, other excimer lasers can scan a smaller laser spot over a large area of the cornea, accomplishing a similar large area ablation.

Because of these unique qualities, the 193 nm excimer laser can be used to meticulously etch large areas of the corneal surface while minimizing damage to remaining tissue.[20,32] PTK is thus a refined methodology of superficial keratectomy.

Wound Healing

Although there appears to be relatively little "collateral" damage to the corneal tissue with excimer laser treatment, corneal wound healing is still important in the surgical outcome. In particular, in the case of PTK where dis-

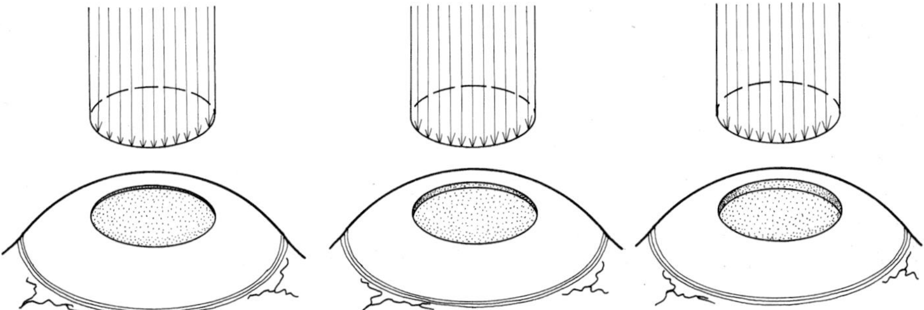

Figure 1–5.   Scheme depicting corneal ablation by the excimer laser beam. An approximately 0.25 1m disc of tissue is removed with each laser pulse. Successive pulses lead to deeper tissue removal.

eased corneas are treated, efficacy of re-epithelialization over the ablated area is important (Fig. 1–6).[33] Moreover, new collagen synthesis is found in the superficial stroma in the area of photoablation (Fig. 1–7).[34] Such wound healing may affect topography and refractive changes after the procedure (see Chapter 6).

With any laser radiation, in particular in the ultraviolet spectrum, there is always concern of the potential for mutagenesis or carcinogenesis. A number of studies have been performed and have shown that the 193 nm excimer laser is neither mutagenic nor carcinogenic.[33,34] This may be in part a result of shielding of the nucleus by the cell's cytoplasm.

Conclusions

The excimer laser in corneal surgery has unique tissue ablation properties. The laser, by removing small amounts of tissue with little concomitant damage to adjacent cornea presents a valuable new tool to the corneal surgeon. As will be seen, a knowledge of the mechanism and effect of excimer laser tissue removal is important in properly selecting patients and in successfully performing the PTK procedure.

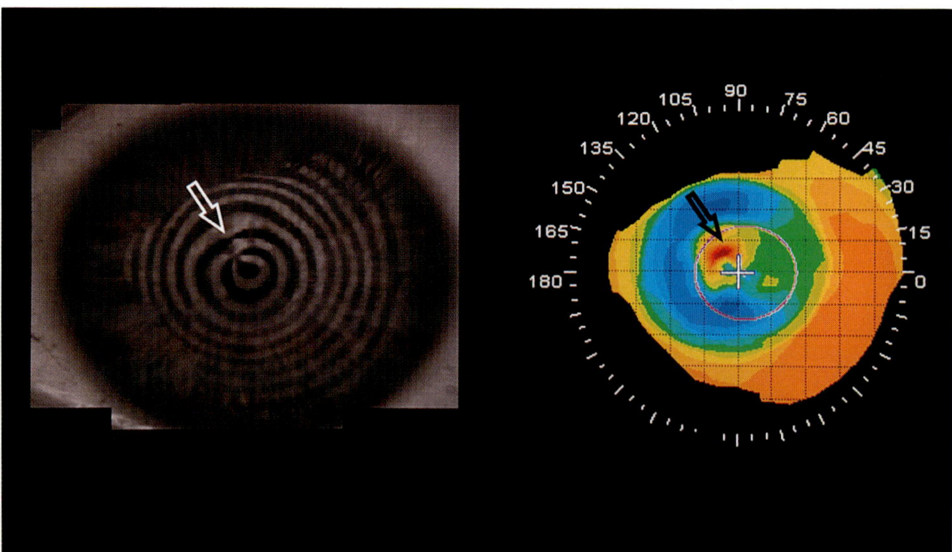

Figure 1–6.   (Left) Placebo disc image in early healing phase following excimer laser treatment shows irregularity of the epithelium leading to **(Right)** a central island pattern on computer-assisted videokeratography.

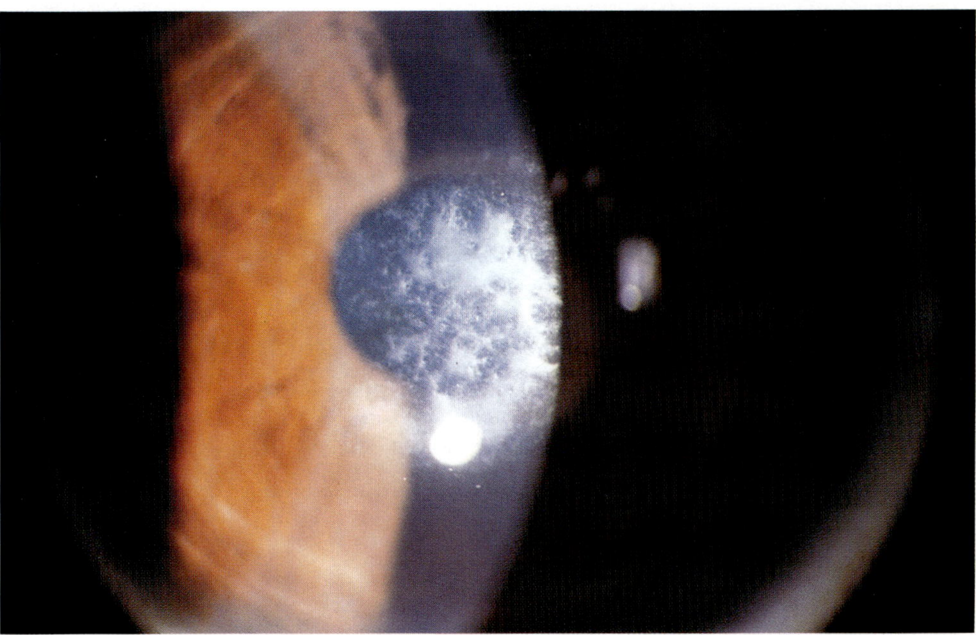

Figure 1–7. Unusual corneal haze and scarring following excimer laser treatment.

References

1. Deutsch TF, Geis MW. Self-developing UV photoresist using excimer laser exposure. J Appl Phys 1983;54:7201–7204.
2. Koren G, Yeh JT. Emission spectra, surface quality, and mechanism of excimer laser radiation. Appl Phys Lett 1984;44:1112.
3. Srinivasan R, Leigh WJ. Ablative photodecompensation on poly(ethylene terephthalate) films. J Am Chem Soc 1982;104:6784.
4. Srinivasan R, Mayne-Bayton V. Self-developing photoetching of poly(ethylene terephthalatate) films by far-ultraviolet excimer laser radiation. Appl Phys Lett 1983;41:576–578.
5 Steinert RF, Puliafito CA. Excimer laser phototherapeutic keratectomy for a corneal nodule. Refract Corneal Surg 1990;6:352.
6. Sher NA, Bowers RA, Zabel RW et al. Clinical use of the 193-nm excimer laser in the treatment of corneal scars. Arch Ophthalmol 1991;109:491–498.
7. Stark WJ, Chamon W. Clinical follow-up of 193 nm ArF excimer laser photokeratectomy. Ophthalmology 1992;99:805–812.
8. Rapuano CJ, Laibson PR. Excimer laser phototherapeutic keratectomy for anterior corneal pathology. CLAO J 1994;20:253–257.
9. Tuunanen TH, Tervo TM. Excimer laser phototherapeutic keratectomy for corneal diseases: a follow-up study. CLAO J 1995;21:67–72.
10. Hersh PS, Kenyon KR. Dystrophies, degnerations, and dysgeneses of the cornea. In Jakobiec F, Albert D (eds): Principles and Practice of Ophthalmology. Philadelphia: WB Saunders, 1993.
11. Hersh PS. Ophthalmic Surgical Procedures. Boston: Little, Brown & Co. 1988:221–225.
12. Trokel S I, Srinivasan R, Braren R. Excimer laser surgery of the cornea. Am J Ophthalmol 1983;96:710–715.
13. L'Esperance FA, Taylor DM, Warner JW. Human excimer laser keratectomy: short term histopathology. J Refract Surg 1988;4:118–124.

14. Marshall J, Trokel SL, Rothery S, Krueger RR. Long-term healing of the central cornea after photorefractive keratectomy using an excimer laser. Ophthalmology 1988;95:1411–1421.
15. Goodman GL, Trokel SL, Stark WJ et al., Corneal healing following laser refractive keratectomy. Arch Ophthalmol 1989;107:1799–1803.
16. Wu WCS, Stark WJ, Green WR. Corneal wound healing excimer laser keratectomy. Arch Ophthalmol 1991;109:1426–1432.
17. Gartry D, Muir MK, Marshall J. Excimer laser treatment of corneal surface pathology; a laboratory and clinical study. Br J Ophthalmol 1991;75:258–268.
18. Rhodes CK. Excimer Lasers. 2nd Ed. New York: Springer, 1984.
19. Burlamacchi P. Laser sources. In Hillenkamp F, Pratesi R, Sacchi CA, eds. Lasers in Biology and Medicine. New York: Plenum, 1980:1–16.
20. Puliafito CA, Steinert RF, Deutsch TF, Hillenkamp F, Dehm EJ, Adler CM. Excimer laser ablation of the cornea and lens: experimental studies. Ophthalmology 1985;92–98:741–748.
21. Dehm EJ, Puliafito CA, Adler CM, Steinert RF. Corneal endothelial injury in rabbits following excimer laser ablation at 193 and 248 nm. Arch Ophthalmol 1986;104:1364–1368.
22. Garrison BJ, Srinivasan R. Microscopic model for the ablative photodecompensation of polymers by far ultraviolet radiation (193 nm). Appl Phys Lett 1984;44:849.
23. Jellinek HH, Srinivasan R. Theory of etching of polymers by far-ultraviolet, high-intensity pulsed laser and long-term irradiation. J Phys Chem 1984;88:3048.
24. Kahle G, Stadter H, Seiler T, Wollensak J. Gas chromatograph/mass spectrometer analysis of excimer and erbium-YAG laser ablated human corneas. Invest Ophthalmol Vis Sci 1992;33:2180–2184.
25. Dyer PE, Al-Dhahir RH. Transient photoacoustic studies of laser tissue ablation. SPIE Proc 1990;1202:46–60.
26. Krueger RR, Trokel SL, Schubert HD. Interaction of ultraviolet laser light with the cornea. Invest Ophthalmol Vis Sci 1985;26:1455–1464.
27. Krueger RR, Trokel SL. Quantitation of corneal ablation by ultraviolet laser light. Arch Ophthalmol 1985;103:1341–1342.
28. Seiler T, Kriegerowski M, Schnoy N, Bende T. Ablation rate of human corneal epithelium and Bowman's layer with the excimer laser (193 nm). J Refract Corneal Surg 1990;6:99–102.
29. McDonald MB, Frantz JM, Klyce SD et al. One year refractive results of central photorefractive keratectomy for myopia in the nonhuman primate cornea. Arch Ophthalmol 1990;108:40–47.
30. Gottsch JD, Rencs EV, Cambier JL, Hall D, Azar DT, Stark WJ. Excimer laser calibration system. J Refract Surg 1996;12:401–411.
31. Puliafito CA, Stern D, Krueger RR, Mandel ER. High-speed photography of excimer laser ablation of the human cornea. Arch Ophthalmol 1987;105:1255.
32. Trokel SL, Srinivasan R, Braren B. Excimer laser surgery of the cornea. Am J Ophthalmol 1983;96:710.
33. Tuft SJ, Zabel RW, Marshall J. Corneal repair following keratectomy: a comparison between conventional surgery and laser photoablation. Invest Ophthalmol Vis Sci 1989;30:1769–1777.
34. Malley DS, Steinert RF, Puliafito CA, Dobi ET. Immunofluorescence study of corneal wound healing after excimer laser anterior keratectomy in the monkey eye. Arch Ophthalmol 1990;108:1316–1322.

2

Case Selection and Surgical Decision Making

Superficial keratectomy, whether mechanical or laser, is the surgical removal of subepithelial fibrous membranes or anterior corneal opacities that occur as a result of corneal degenerative and dystrophic conditions, infections, and other causes.[1-4]

The efficacy of PTK in particular seems to be related to several factors, including the tissue ablation properties of the laser (see Chapter 1), the nature of the preoperative corneal disorder and consequent treatment strategy (see Chapter 3), the patient's subjective complaint, and the preoperative refractive error (see Chapter 6). Careful attention should be directed toward the specific patient complaints to better determine if PTK may be expected to achieve the desired clinical goals. An in-depth history and careful consideration of the individual patient's needs, thus, is essential. For instance, a patient with Salzmann's nodules, while having good visual acuity, may complain of recalcitrant monocular diplopia and photophobia, and PTK may be rewarded by resolution of the patient's subjective complaints. Another patient may complain of poor visual acuity as a consequence of Reis-Buckler's dystrophy. However, a hyperopic refractive error in this patient may make PTK undesirable.

An understanding of the indications for PTK, surgical goals, and potential results is important to properly select cases. The surgeon should realize that PTK is not the treatment of choice for all anterior corneal pathology. This chapter therefore details the parameters that must be understood to determine which treatment is best for patients with superficial corneal disorders.

Manual Versus Laser-Assisted Superficial Keratectomy

A comparison of the relative advantages and disadvantages of manual superficial keratectomy vs. PTK is presented in Table 2–1.

Manual superficial keratectomy is particularly applicable for disorders of the epithelium and subepithelial–basement membrane zone, where manual removal of pathology is technically easy and is not associated with significant postoperative scarring. It is also useful for somewhat deeper disorders if the pathology can be resected without significantly disturbing Bowman's layer and producing postoperative scarring.[1–16] Manual superficial keratectomy has been successfully utilized for epithelial basement membrane dystrophy,[2,11,14] Reis-Buckler's dystrophy,[2,7,9] granular dystrophy,[2,5] "proud nebulae" or superficial corneal scarring in keratoconus,[2,6] vernal shield ulcers,[12] squamous cell carcinoma,[2] anterior corneal pannus of aniridia,[2] secondary amyloidosis,[2] Salzmann's nodular degeneration,[2,10] and band keratopathy.[2,15,16]

In the largest series to date, Gangadhar et al.[2] reported 200 cases successfully treated with manual superficial keratectomy with improvement in visual acuity or comfort, depending on the preoperative indications. Repeat procedures for recurrent pathology had similar results. Only three major complications were reported: Two eyes developed anterior stromal scarring following removal of band keratopathy, and one eye developed microbial keratitis following removal of an apical keratoconus nodule.

In contrast, PTK may be performed on a wide spectrum of superficial corneal and anterior stromal disorders.[17–50] The spectrum of pathology includes all of those amenable to manual superficial keratectomy, plus those in which the pathology cannot be safely or effectively removed manually. As such, it is an alternative to lamellar or penetrating keratoplasty in anterior corneal disorders that cannot be resected by simple manual techniques. In addition, the PTK procedure does not appear to influence the efficacy of

Table 2–1   Manual Versus Phototherapeutic Superficial Keratectomy

MANUAL	PHOTOTHERAPEUTIC
Inexpensive	Expensive
Simple equipment	Complex equipment
Technically easy	Variable level of difficulty
May be repeated often	May be repeated, but risk of hyperopia
No change in spherical power	Hyperopic shift
Little risk for iatrogenic irregular astigmatism	May induce irregular astigmatism
Some pathology, especially anterior stromal, not amenable to treatment	Effective ablation of Bowman's layer and anterior stroma

subsequent keratoplasty if necessary. Thus, it is a safe procedure to attempt even in the case where subsequent keratoplasty may still be necessary.

PTK has been reported in the successful management of recurrent erosion syndromes due to trauma or epithelial basement membrane dystrophy,[20,22,29,30] persistent epithelial defects,[22] superficial corneal scarring,[22,25,27] Salzmann's nodular degeneration,[28] Reis-Buckler's dystrophy,[19,27,32,34,38] granular dystrophy,[19] lattice dystrophy,[19] band keratopathy,[22,27,36] apical scarring or "proud nebulae" of keratoconus,[22,35] and climatic droplet keratopathy.[17] As with manual keratectomy, it has also been applied successfully to recurrent disease, including recurrent dystrophy in grafts with lattice or granular dystrophy[38,51] and epithelial basement membrane dystrophy.[20,22,29]

An important principle to understand before attempting PTK is that the excimer laser, by virtue of its unique tissue ablation properties (see Chapter 1), reproduces the topography "it sees."[44,48] Elimination of corneal opacification but retention of an irregular anterior contour will have no impact on pre-existing irregular astigmatism. On the other hand, irregular ablation of previously normal corneal stroma due to differential ablation rates of normal and pathological tissue may iatrogenically induce irregular astigmatism. In addition, ablation of the anterior corneal stroma may flatten the corneal curvature, inducing a net hyperopic shift, which becomes more significant with progressively deeper treatment (see Chapter 6).[17,19,22,34,36,44,49,50] Other potential complications of excimer PTK are discussed in Chapters 5 and 6.[19,47,50–55]

Modifications of the surgical technique may reduce, but not completely eliminate, the complications associated with exact anatomical reproduction of the anterior corneal contour, induction of irregular astigmatism, and hyperopic shifts.[43,44,48] It is these potential technical difficulties that prohibit the unrestricted use of PTK in the management of all anterior corneal pathology and require careful evaluation of the anticipated outcome before offering this procedure to the patient.[1,56]

Fortunately, several modifications of excimer laser technique can minimize these problems (see Chapters 3 and 6). Briefly, the technique of "masking" with selective debridement of the epithelium and the use of viscous fluids that absorb the laser energy to "protect the valleys and expose the peaks" may result in an improved final corneal contour.[43–45,48] Hyperopic shifts can be reduced by minimizing the ablation of the anterior corneal stroma, "peripheral blending" of the edge of the treatment zone, or by gently rocking the patient's head and "polishing" during the laser treatment.[41,43]

Case Selection

The advent of phototherapeutic ablation capabilities has expanded the indications of superficial keratectomy to the more difficult to resect anterior

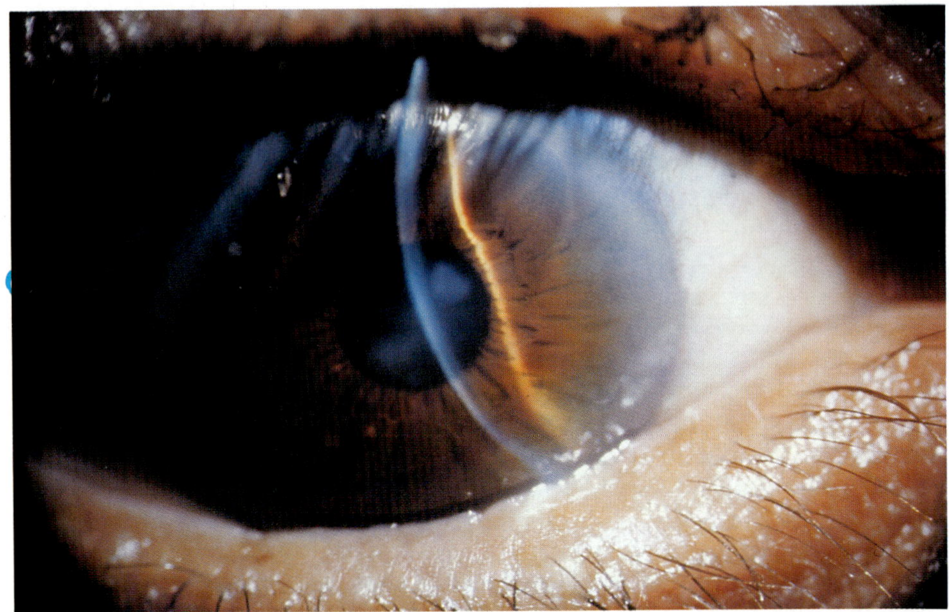

A

Figure 2–1.   Salzmann's nodular degeneration. **(A)** Isolated corneal nodules in the optical zone produce mild foreign body sensation, occasional recurrent erosion syndrome, and mild visual acuity disturbance due to irregular astigmatism. Appropriate treatment is by manual superficial keratectomy. *(Continued on following page)*

corneal lesions, but does not make it the procedure of choice in every anterior corneal disorder. It is important to understand that:

1. The primary diagnosis does not necessarily dictate the treatment of choice, since various clinical presentations of the same disorder may dictate different therapeutic approaches (Fig. 2–1).
2. Identical clinical presentation does not dictate the treatment of choice, since functional requirements of the patient may also require different therapeutic approaches. For example, Reis-Buckler's dystrophy in a myopic eye may be successfully treated with PTK. However, the same situation may suggest only manual superficial keratectomy in a hyperopic eye.

Therapeutic Parameters

Appropriate recommendations regarding the treatment of choice can be made only after analyzing the horizontal and vertical distribution and pattern of the pathology, the applicability of manual and phototherapeutic techniques, and the functional objectives of treatment.

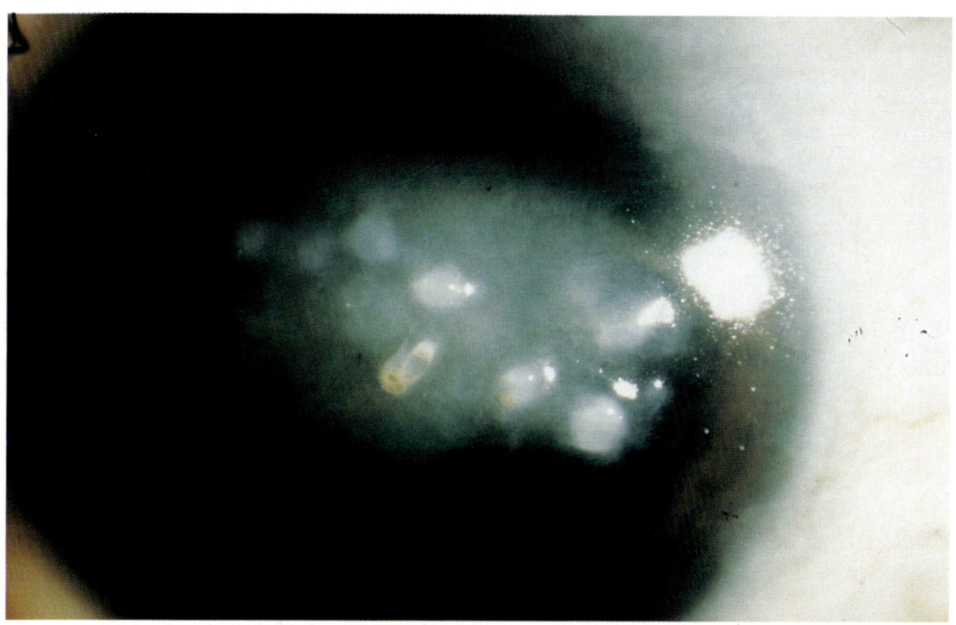

B

Figure 2–1 (B).   Advanced, confluent nodules in optical zone with anterior stromal scarring is profoundly disturbing visual function, as well as producing disabling recurrent epithelial erosions. Successful treatment will require a combined approach of manual excision of the superficial nodules and phototherapeutic keratectomy of the pathology at Bowman's layer and in the anterior corneal stroma.

Horizontal Assessment

Corneal pathology can be categorized horizontally into the optical, paracentral, and peripheral zone. For purposes of surgical decision making, the classification is based on the most central area of involvement.

The *optical zone* is defined as the central 3–4 mm, where pathology may directly (through clouding of visual axis) or indirectly (through the induction of irregular astigmatism) diminish visual function. Treatment by either manual or phototherapeutic keratectomy in this region may produce permanent alterations in visual function by inducing changes in corneal clarity or contour. Examples of disorders in this zone amenable to superficial keratectomy include epithelial basement membrane dystrophy, Meesman's dystrophy, Reis-Buckler's dystrophy, band keratopathy, climatic droplet keratopathy, postinfectious and post-pterygium scarring, the anterior variants of granular and lattice dystrophy, and recurrent dystrophies.

The *paracentral zone* is defined as the midperipheral zone, where pathology may indirectly affect visual function by the induction of irregular astigmatism or glare. More often, however, treatment for disorders in this region is considered for recurrent epithelial erosions or potential extension into the

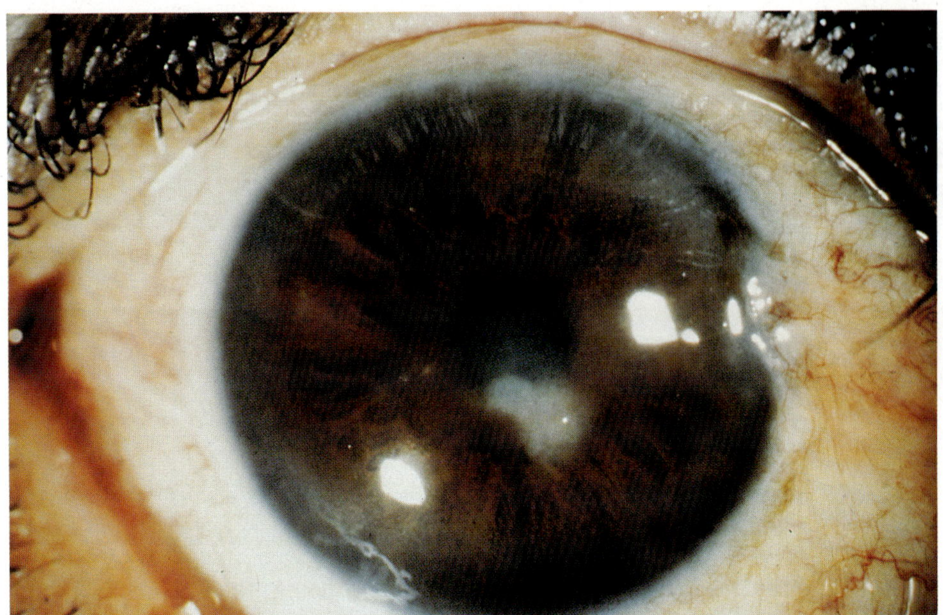

Figure 2–2. Paracentral corneal pathology. Any visual disturbance produced by these lesions will be due to irregular astigmatism, not to disturbance of media clarity. **(A)** Isolated Salzmann's nodule, just outside the visual axis. Therapeutic objectives can be achieved by manual excision. The additional potential clarity at the level of Bowman's that may be achieved with PTK does not enhance the final functional result and risks potential alteration of the contour of Bowman's layer in the adjacent pupillary zone with permanent, detrimental effect on visual function. *(Continued on following page)*

visual axis. Treatment by manual superficial keratectomy in this zone poses little risk to the visual axis. PTK in this region may produce alterations in visual function due to iatrogenic changes in the contour of adjacent corneal tissue in the visual axis. Although it is unusual to see pathology localized specifically to this area, Salzmann's nodules (Fig. 2–2A), post-traumatic epithelial–basement membrane disorders, and postinfectious scars (Fig. 2–2B) may occur here. In addition, many types of pathology gradually encroach on the visual axis from the paracentral zone, including pterygium, band keratopathy, and climatic droplet keratopathy.

The *peripheral zone* has little or no direct impact on visual function. Similarly, treatment with either manual or PTK will have little adverse impact on the visual axis. Anterior disorders that are considered for keratectomy in this region include pterygium, post-traumatic corneal epithelial erosions, postinfectious scars, and peripheral degenerations such as climatic droplet keratopathy (Fig. 2–3).

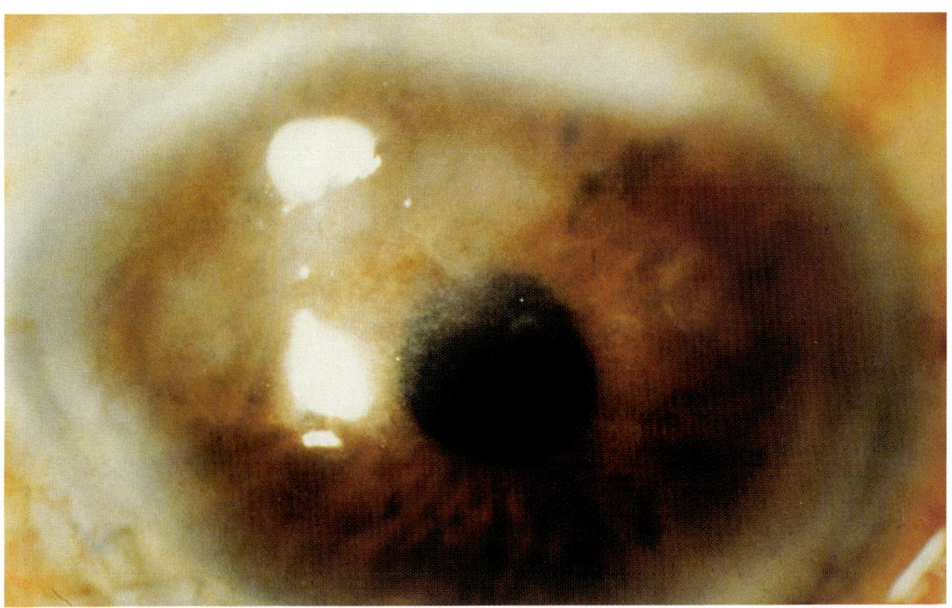

Figure 2–2 (B).   Postinfectious corneal scarring that spares the visual axis, but is producing mild glare symptoms. This lesion is not inducing epithelial irregularity and, therefore, does not substantially decrease visual acuity. Manual excision is not technically feasible, leaving PTK as the only superficial surgical option. The risk of induction of irregular astigmatism due to off-center ablation, however, does not justify the minimal benefits of slight reduction of glare.

Pattern Assessment

After horizontal assessment, corneal disorders in the visual axis may then be classified by the pattern of distribution as *nodular, segmental, diffuse,* or *complete* (Fig. 2–4).

Nodular pathology refers to well-circumscribed lesions that are single or few in number and surrounded by normal cornea. For such disorders, manual superficial keratectomy may be performed without disturbing the normal, contiguous cornea. PTK may be more effective in completely removing difficult lesions and result in less postoperative scarring, but it is much more likely to alter normal, contiguous corneal tissue and induce irregular astigmatism. Examples of nodular pathology include Salzmann's nodular degeneration, the so-called proud nebula or superficial scar tissue in longterm rigid contact lens wearers with keratoconus (Fig. 2–5A), and postinfectious scarring.

Segmental lesions are functionally similar to nodular lesions, but occupy a greater percentage of the optical zone. Still, they are associated with normal

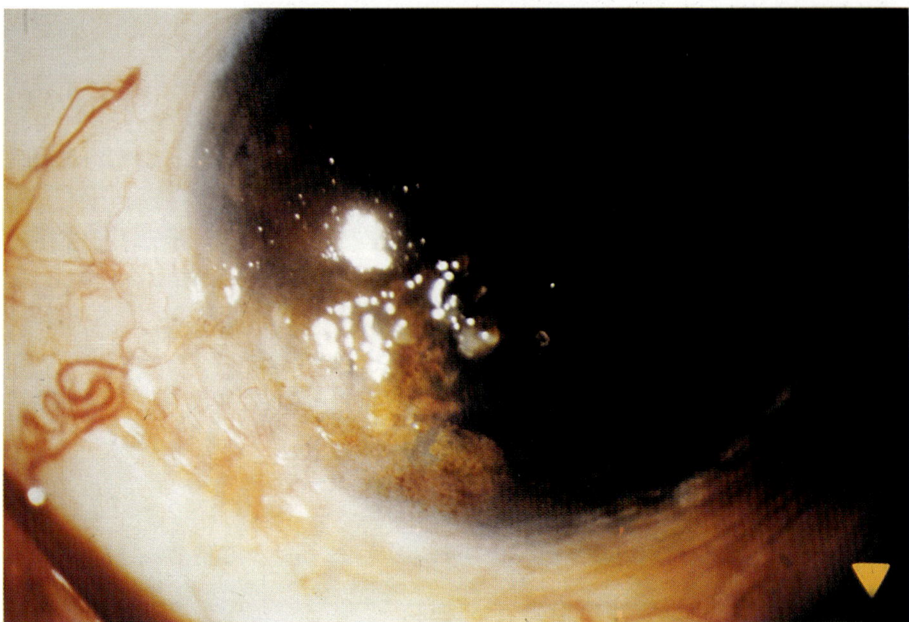

Figure 2–3.   Peripheral corneal pathology. Secondary climatic droplet keratopathy has occurred in the area of previous corneal infiltrate, with persistent foreign body sensation and recurrent erosions. Simple manual excision of the superficial pathology is all that is required to restore comfort, but there are no absolute contraindications for using PTK in this case.

adjacent tissue that is vulnerable to unwanted laser ablation. Examples include pterygium extending into the visual axis (Fig. 2–5B), residual post-pterygium or postinfectious scarring, band keratopathy, and climatic droplet keratopathy encroaching on the visual axis.

Diffuse lesions are symmetrically present throughout the optical zone, but do not occupy the entire surface area. Usually it is necessary to remove the entire plane in which the pathology lies to accomplish the therapeutic objectives. Examples of diffuse lesions are epithelial membrane dystrophy, post-traumatic basement membrane disorders, Meesman's dystrophy, and anterior stromal dystrophies such as granular (Fig. 2–5C) or lattice dystrophy.

Complete lesions are continuously present throughout the entire surface area of the optical zone. Disorders that present with this pattern include band keratopathy, Reis-Buckler's dystrophy (Fig. 2–5D), and climatic droplet keratopathy.

Vertical Assessment

The vertical level of involvement of corneal disorders is divided into (1) pre-Bowman's layer, (2) Bowman's layer, (3) anterior stromal, and (4) stromal

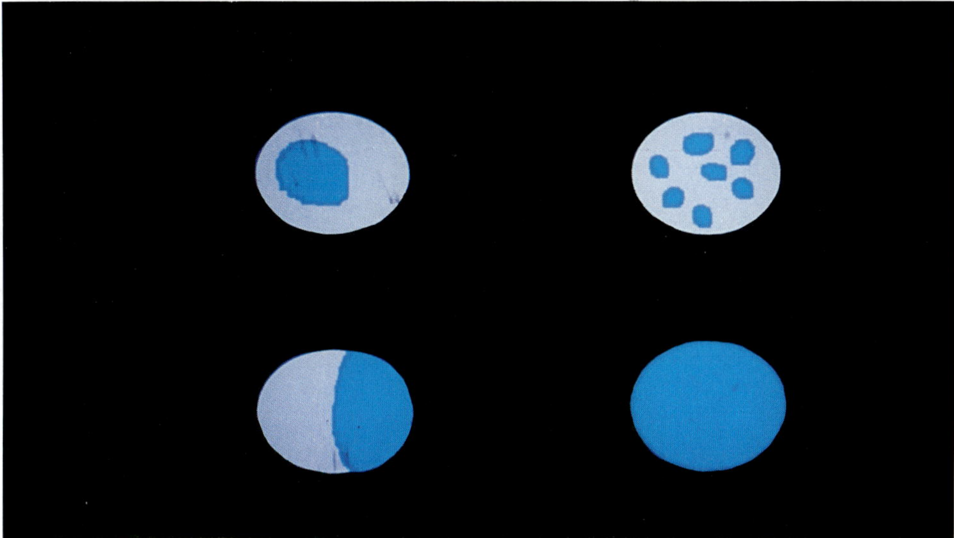

Figure 2–4. Schematic depiction of the four patterns of distribution of pathology in the optical zone: nodular **(Upper left)**, segmental, **(Lower left)** diffuse, **(Upper right)** and complete **(Lower right)**. (Reproduced with permission from Wagoner.[1])

Figure 2–5. *(Following two pages)* Clinical examples of the four patterns of distribution of pathology in the optical zone. **(A)** Nodular. A subepithelial nodule or "proud nebula" in an eye with long-standing keratoconus and hard contact lens wear. Removal of the nodule by either manual or phototherapeutic keratectomy is likely to restore contact lens tolerance. Because the lesion is well circumscribed and easily resectable by manual techniques, phototherapeutic removal with its concomitant risk of alteration of adjacent cornea is probably not advised. **(B)** Segmental. A pterygium with scarring that is approaching the visual axis is easily resectable by manual techniques, although some anterior stromal scarring may persist in the nasal segment of the optical zone. Management of the persistent scarring by PTK should be avoided, if possible, due to risk of inducing alteration of the unaffected portions of the optical zone. **(C)** Diffuse. Extensive involvement of the central optical zone with granular dystrophy. Although a final decision on the treatment of choice must also take into account the depth of the lesions and therapeutic objectives (relief of recurrent epithelial erosions or improved visual acuity), PTK will probably be required to obtain an optimal result. The impact of ablation of clear areas of cornea between the lesions can be minimized by a well-centered ablation utilizing fluid-masking techniques and peripheral blending or "head rocking" maneuvers to minimize undesirable hyperopic shifts. **(D)** Complete. Reis-Buckler's dystrophy is a classic example of complete involvement of Bowman's layer in the optical zone with pathology that is easily resectable by either manual or phototherapeutic keratectomy. The final decision is contingent on the desired spherical refractive outcome and depth of the pathology.

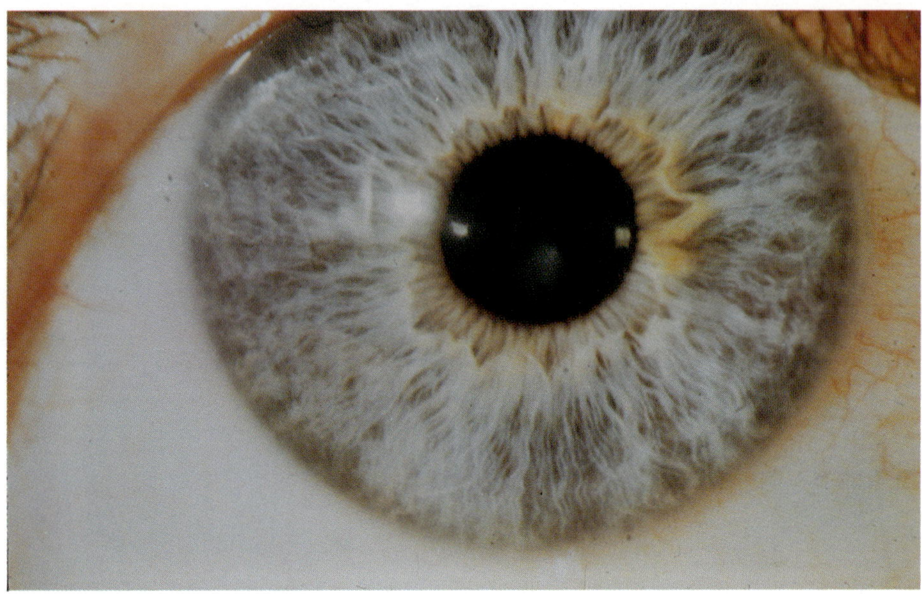

Figure 2–5 (A)

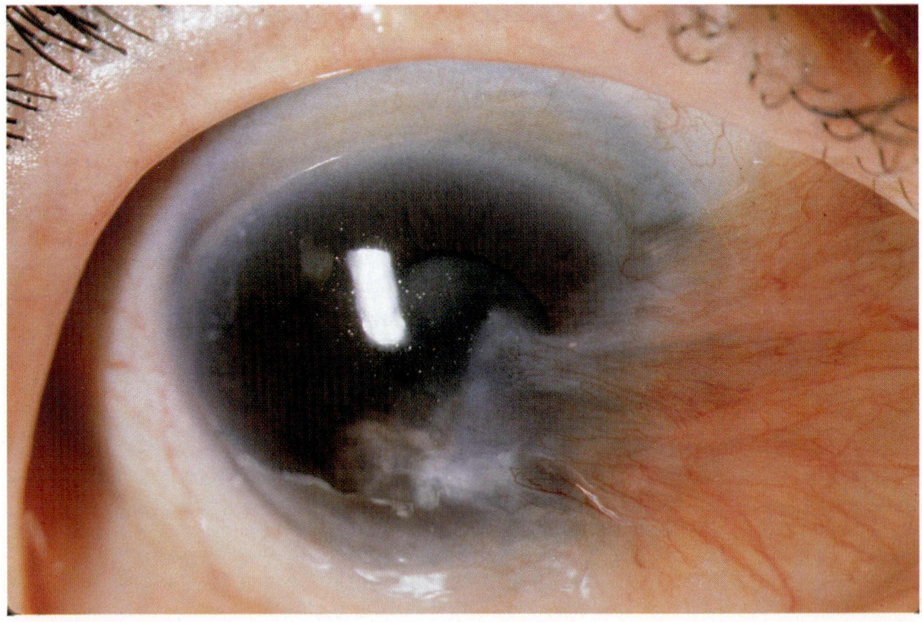

Figure 2–5 (B)

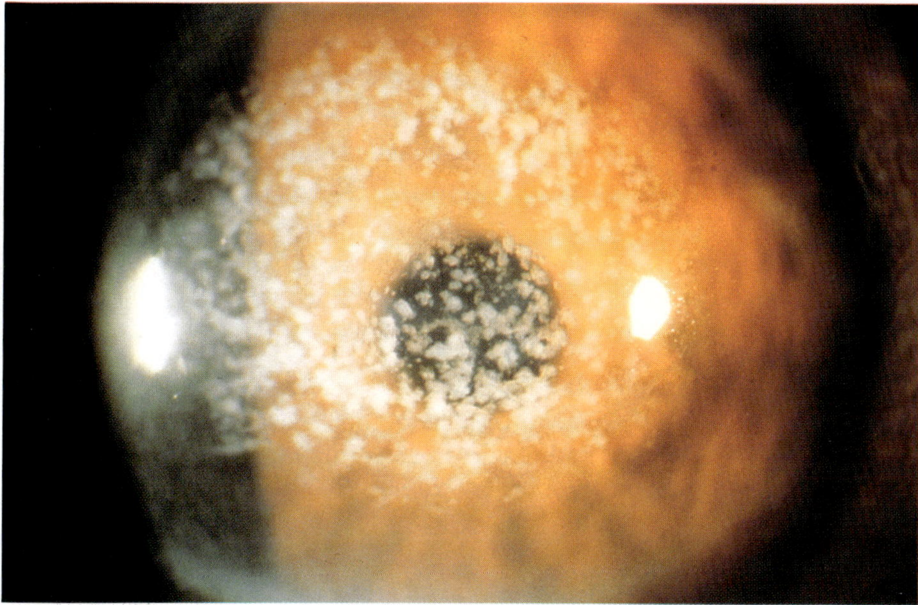

Figure 2–5 (C)

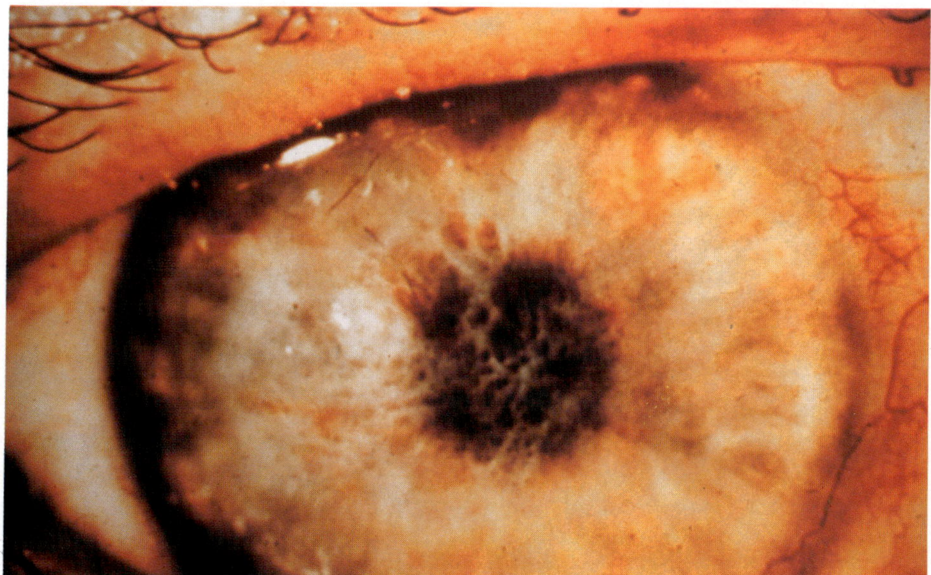

Figure 2–5 (D)

(Fig. 2–6). The depth is defined as the most posterior extension of the pathology *intended* for resection. For example, lattice dystrophy may involve full thickness of stroma, but if superficial keratectomy is being performed for recurrent erosions and irregular astigmatism, the depth of involvement is classified as anterior stromal. If the stromal pathology is the major contributor to decreased vision, and the stromal deposits must be addressed to improve visual function, then the pathology is considered stromal.

Pre-Bowman's refers to disorders that involve the epithelium and basement membrane zone, but completely spare Bowman's layer. This may include primary or secondary epithelial basement membrane disorders (Fig. 2–7A).

Bowman's refers to all pathology incorporated into Bowman's layer, with or without epithelial and epithelial basement membrane involvement. Examples include band keratopathy, Reis-Buckler's dystrophy, postinfectious scarring, and "smooth" climatic droplet keratopathy (Fig. 2–7B).

Anterior stromal refers to pathologic processes that have extended beneath Bowman's layer into the anterior 100–150 µm of the cornea. Examples of disorders in this category include the anterior variants of granular or lattice dystrophy, postinfectious scarring, and "rough" climatic droplet keratopathy (Fig. 2–7C).

Stromal pathology refers to disorders where excision of deep stromal lamellae (>150 µm) is required to achieve the desired visual outcome. Macular

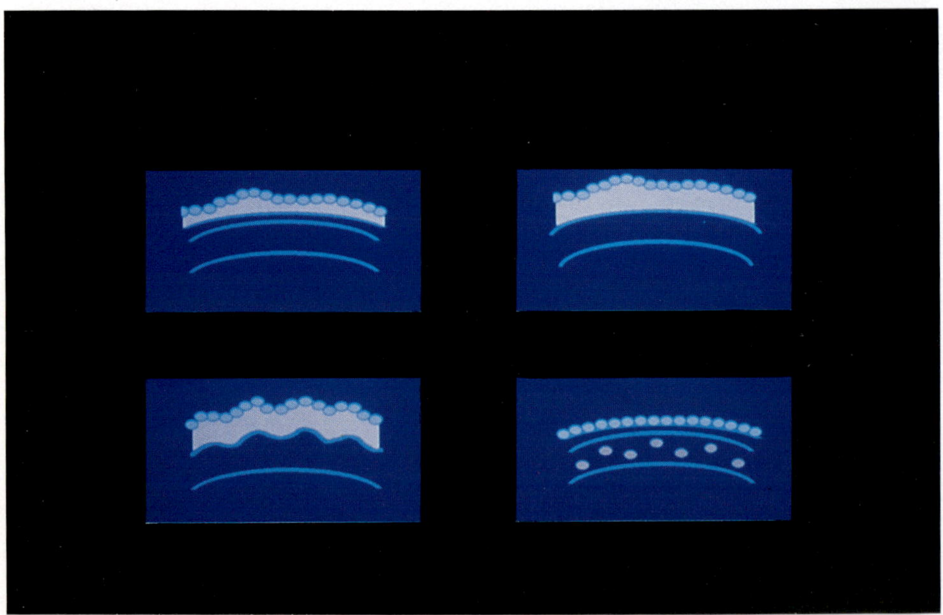

Figure 2–6. Schematic depiction of the four depths of pathology in the optical zone: pre-Bowman's layer, **(Upper left)** Bowman's layer, **(Upper right)** anterior stromal, **(Lower left)** and stromal **(Lower right)**. (Reproduced with permission from Wagoner.[1])

corneal dystrophy (Fig. 2–7D) is an example of a disorder for which neither manual nor phototherapeutic keratectomy is of much value because penetrating keratoplasty is necessary in such cases of deep stromal involvement.

Applicability of Technique

The actual ability of the procedure to accomplish the desired objective of removing the pathologic process must be ascertained. Almost invariably, any disorder amenable to manual resection can be removed by PTK, although the converse is not always the case.

Generally, the more posterior the pathology extends, the more likely manual keratectomy is to be technically less desirable than PTK. At Bowman's layer, disorders such as Reis-Buckler's dystrophy may be easily resectable manually, and disorders like recurrent band keratopathy may be easily resectable in some cases and not others (Fig. 2–8). Other disorders such as superficial corneal scars and anterior corneal dystrophies are typically very difficult to remove manually but are amenable to PTK.

Functional Objectives

The ultimate determinant of the appropriate technique of superficial keratectomy is the functional objective of the procedure.

Visual objectives relate to final visual acuity. In assessing a patient's needs, not only is the final corrected visual acuity important, but any potential adverse alteration in uncorrected visual acuity that may result from undesirable hyperopic shifts must be taken into account.

Nonvisual objectives include reducing the pain associated with recurrent erosion syndromes or other superficial corneal disorders, decreasing optical problems such as glare, halo, or monocular diplopia, or clearing the visual axis for subsequent surgery. For example, PTK may be performed in an eye

Figure 2–7. *(Following two pages)* Clinical examples of the four depths of pathology in the optical zone. **(A)** Pre-Bowman's layer. Epithelial–basement membrane dystrophy is easily resectable by simple epithelial debridement, which is the procedure of choice. PTK is only indicated for intractable recurrent erosions not amenable to debridement or anterior stromal puncture or if concomitant reduction in myopic refractive error is desired. **(B)** Bowman's layer. Climatic droplet keratopathy, smooth variant, is a classic example of pathology that is not easily amenable to manual resection and must be removed by phototherapeutic ablation. **(C)** Anterior stromal. Climatic droplet keratopathy, irregular variant, has superficial globules that can be easily manually resected. Removal of deeper, anterior stromal deposits requires laser ablation with skillful use of masking techniques due to differential ablation rates of the hyaline deposits and normal cornea, as well as pre-existing irregularity of stromal thickness that is almost invariably present. **(D)** Stromal. Disorders such as macular dystrophy where the visual disability is due to full thickness stromal involvement are not effectively treated by either manual or phototherapeutic keratectomy.

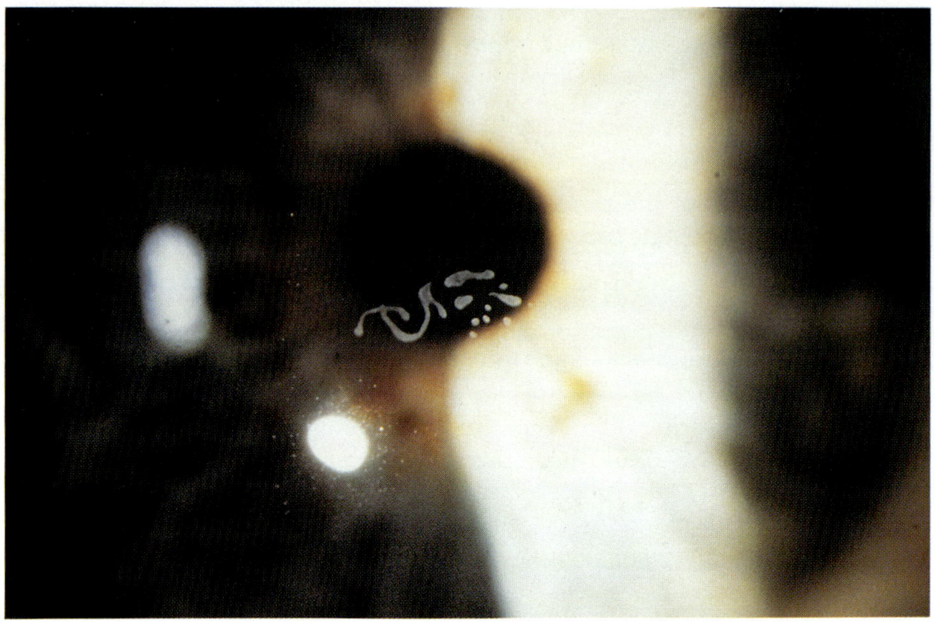

Figure 2–7 (A)

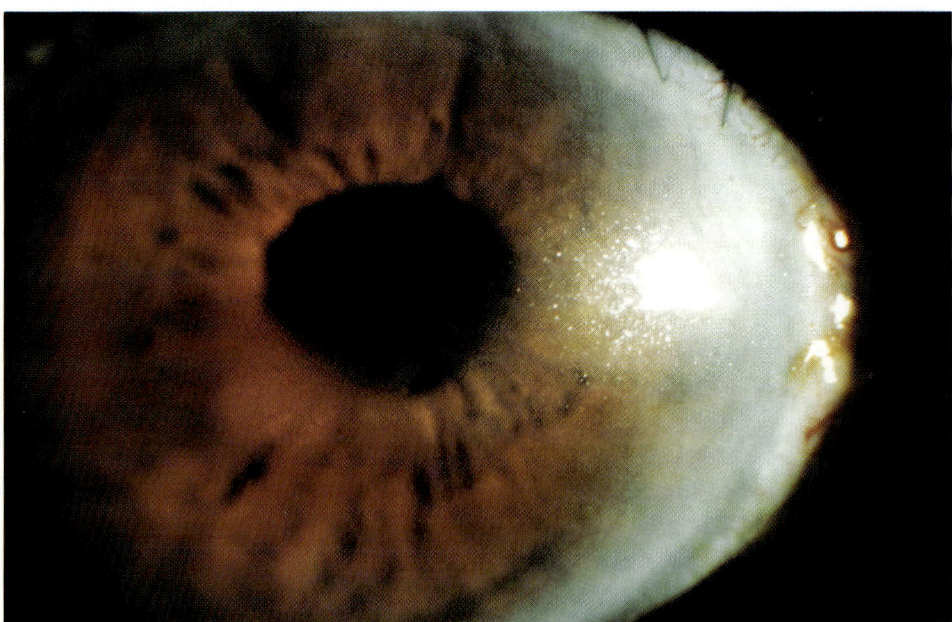

Figure 2–7 (B)

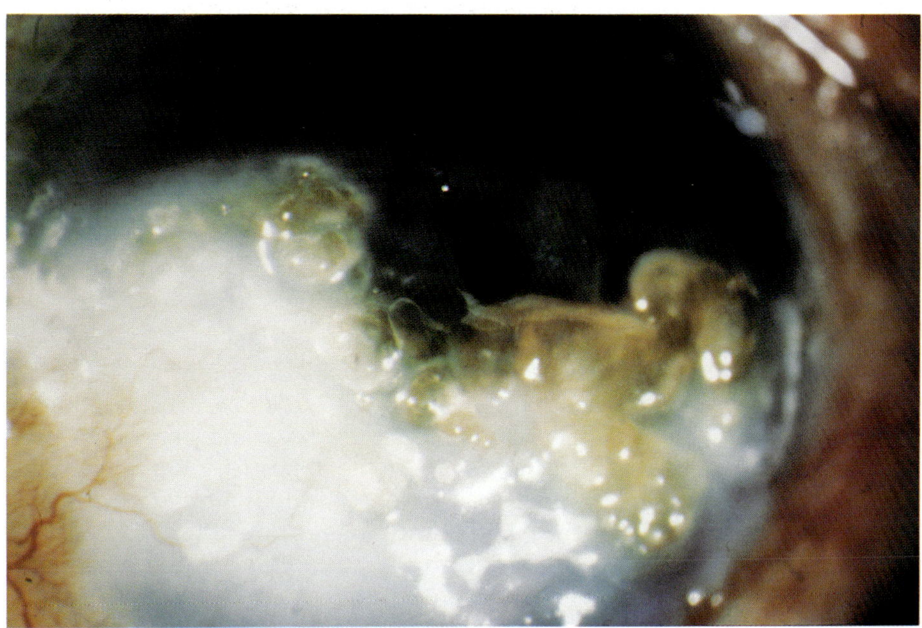

Figure 2–7 (C)

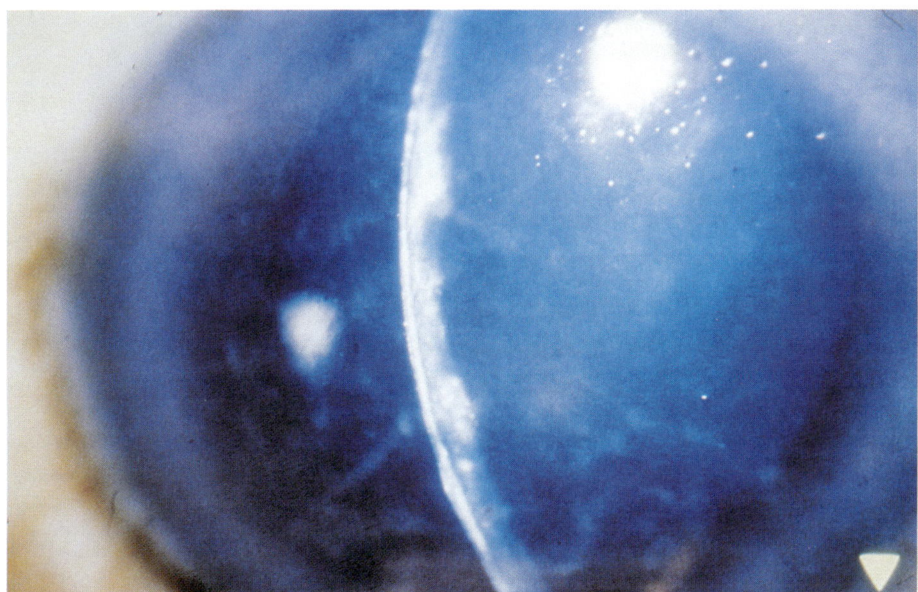

Figure 2–7 (D)

with combined climatic droplet keratopathy and cataract to clear the visualization of the anterior chamber to facilitate subsequent cataract surgery.[17]

Often there will be more than one objective for a particular patient (Fig. 2–9). For instance, Reis-Bucklers' corneal dystrophy may disturb vision secondary to corneal opacification and irregular astigmatism while the patient is suffering discomfort as a result of epithelial dysadherence.

Therapeutic Algorithm

The algorithm presented in Figure 2–10 provides a framework for arriving at the most suitable surgical choice for superficial keratectomy. A color coding (green, red, yellow) system has been devised to allow consideration of PTK (green light) in a manner analogous to the risks and benefits of proceeding through a busy intersection. A green light is usually, but not always, associated with complete safe passage. A yellow caution light indicates that it may be hazardous to proceed, and additional information must be taken into account before proceeding. Generally, a red light is an absolute indication to stop, except in special situations where proceeding can be considered after appropriate considerations of the risk.

The first major trifurcation in the algorithm is into the optical zone, paracentral zone, and peripheral zone. Once pathology is subsumed under one of these categories, the preoperative evaluation will then proceed in a stepwise process consecutively through the pattern assessment, vertical assessment, and functional assessment as depicted in Fig. 2–9. The patient's refractive status must also be considered, as discussed in Chapter 6.

Optical Zone

For pathology in the optical zone, the next step is to determine the pattern of pathology and categorize it as nodular, segmental, diffuse, or complete.

Nodular or *segmental pathology* directly affects visual acuity if it is directly in the visual axis and indirectly by inducing irregular astigmatism if it is slightly eccentric to the visual axis. The functional objective of therapy is usually to excise the pathology to restore a normal anterior corneal contour and avoid altering normal, contiguous cornea. These objectives can usually be easily achieved with manual excision. PTK offers little additional benefit

Figure 2–8. *(Following two pages)* Band keratopathy is a disorder that may or may not be amenable to manual resection with EDTA. **(A,B)** Band keratopathy effectively treated with EDTA scrub, demonstrating remarkable clearing of Bowman's layer. **(C,D)** Band keratopathy in an eye with long-standing intraocular inflammation due to juvenile rheumatoid arthritis shows inadequate clearing of Bowman's layer/anterior stromal opacification after EDTA scrub. PTK may be the appropriate technique in this case.

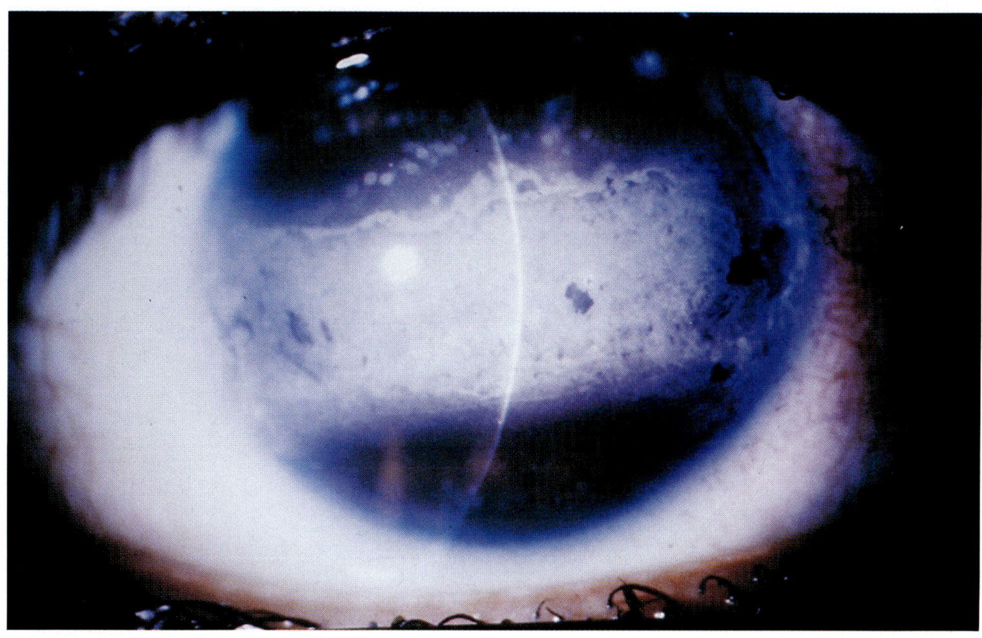

Figure 2–8 (A)

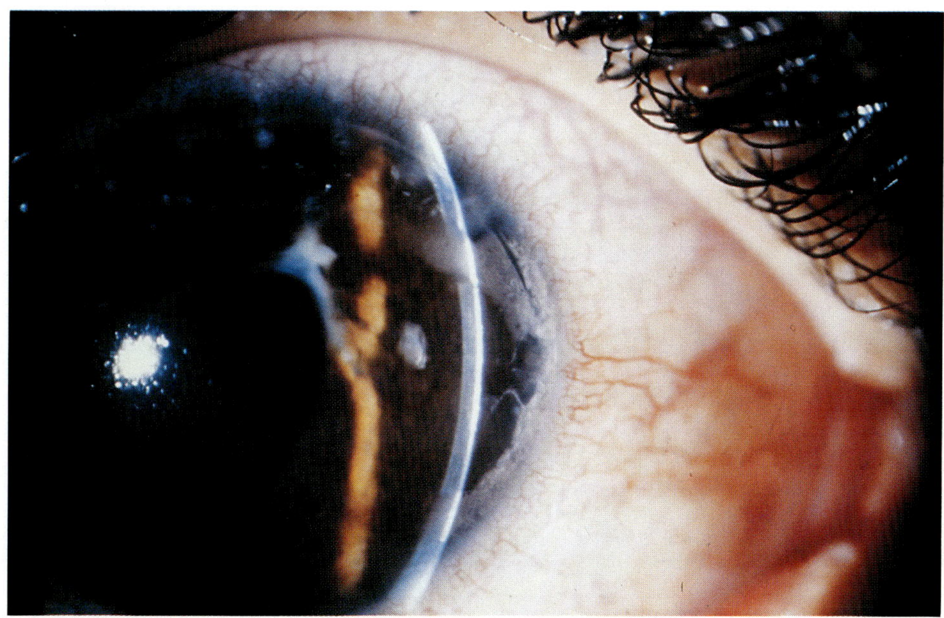

Figure 2–8 (B)

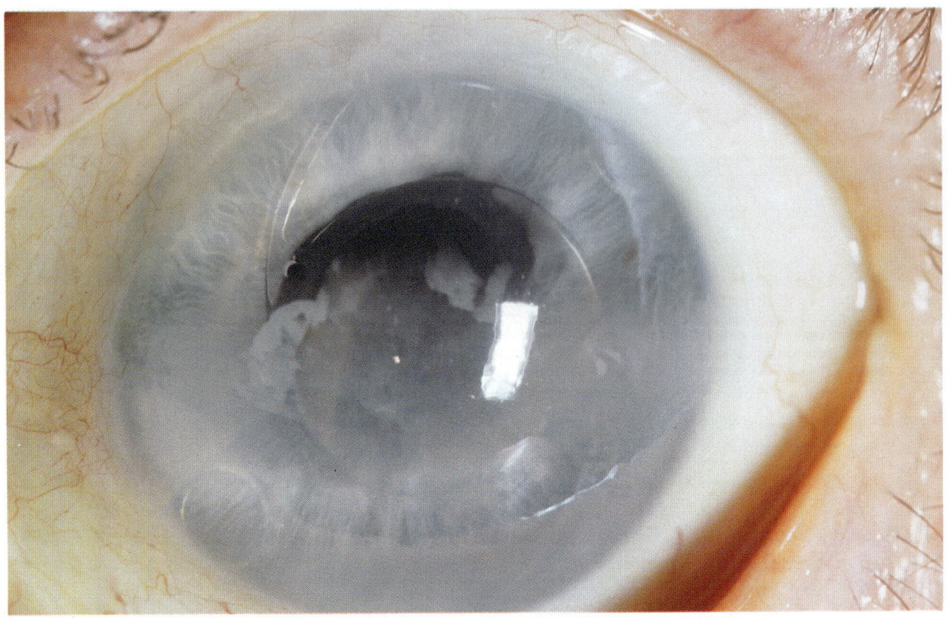

Figure 2–8 (C)

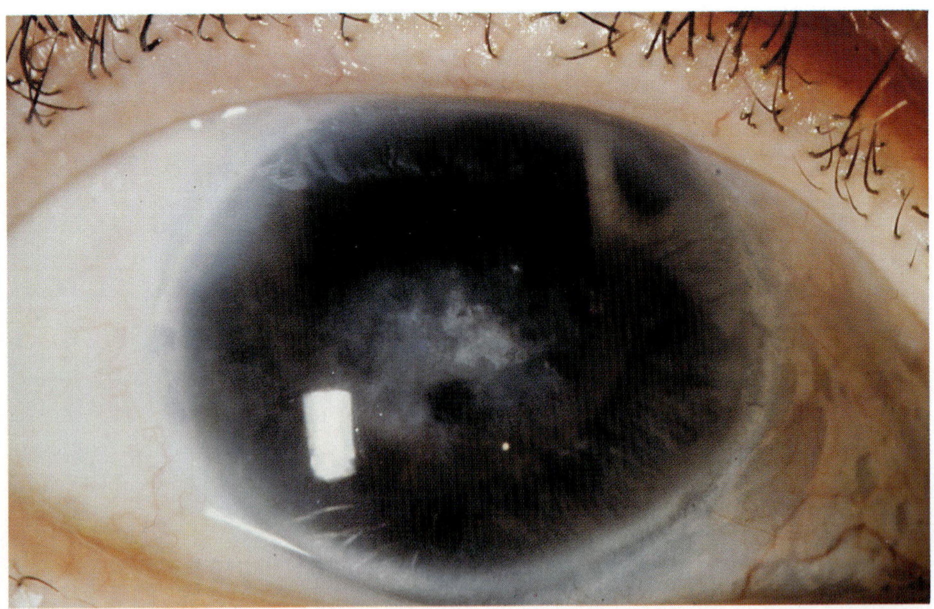

Figure 2–8 (D)

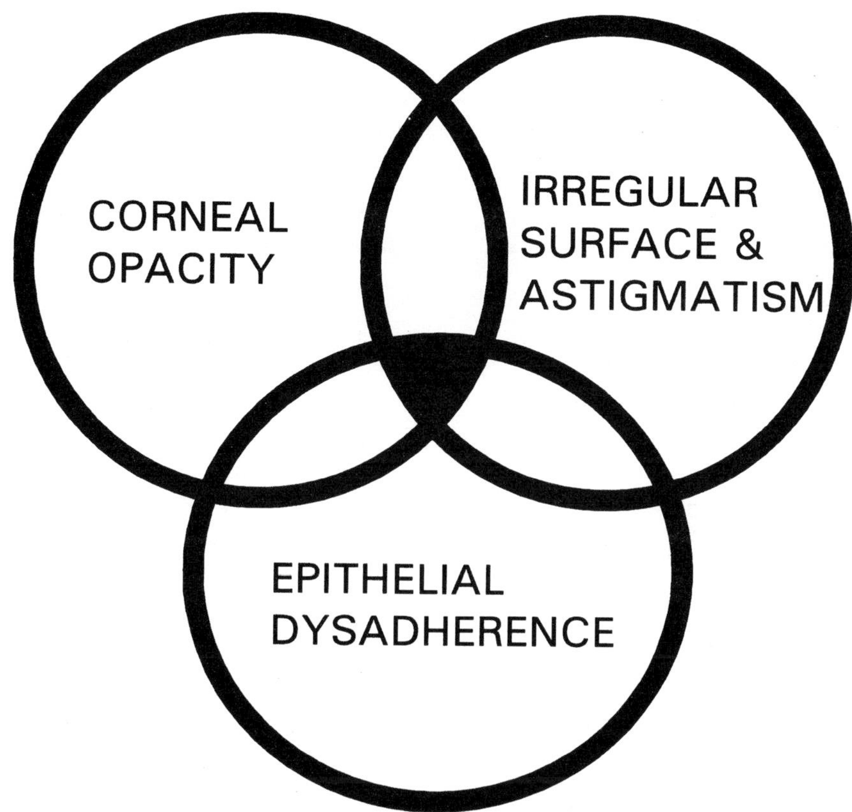

Figure 2–9. Indications for phototherapeutic or superficial keratectomy: (1) Corneal opacity, (2) Irregular corneal surface and astigmatism, (3) Epithelial dysadherence. Such indications may overlap in a number of corneal disease processes.

other than possibly more complete excision of the pathology, although this will be of little therapeutic benefit unless the pathology is directly in the visual axis. Selective photoablation of a dense, focal scar is nearly impossible due to differential ablation rates of the scar and surrounding tissue[50] combined with inability to ensure perfect fluid masking.[48] Also, photoablation of a focal lesion will invariably result in some ablation of contiguous, normal tissue and, for pathology in the optical zone, induce various amounts of irregular astigmatism.

If the pathology is directly in the visual axis, complete excision may be more of a priority than if it is eccentric, especially if the visual effect is due to the density of the scar and it cannot be adequately resected manually. In such cases, phototherapeutic "polishing" may be required for complete excision of visually significant pathology at Bowman's layer or deeper to obtain maximum benefit and minimize induced astigmatism (see Chapter 3).

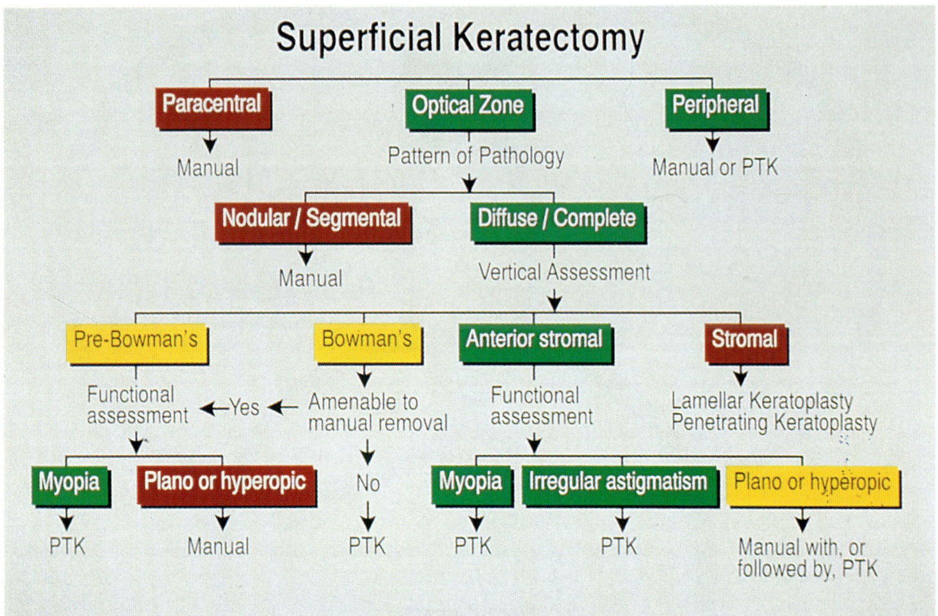

Figure 2–10.   Therapeutic algorithm for surgical decision-making in superficial keratectomy. The algorithm proceeds from top to bottom, taking the following considerations in order: (1) horizontal assessment, (2) pattern assessment, (3) vertical assessment, (4) applicability of the technique, and (5) functional objectives. Green color coding indicates parameters remain favorable for PTK. Red color coding indicates that significant contraindications for PTK exist, and the manual superficial keratectomy is the treatment of choice. Yellow color coding indicates that additional parameters must be considered before a final decision is made, or, if it is at the end of the algorithm, that PTK should be performed with caution. (Reproduced with permission from Wagoner.[1])

Diffuse or *complete pathology* may affect visual function by obstructing the visual axis, as well as inducing irregular astigmatism. Selective removal of individual components of the pathology is often difficult or impossible, and excision of the entire layer of involved cornea (e.g., pre-Bowman's layer for epithelium for map-dot-fingerprint dystrophy, Bowman's layer for band keratopathy) is frequently required. Before making a final decision, additional parameters must be evaluated.

The next step for disorders in the optical zone is the vertical assessment of the depth of the pathology as pre-Bowman's, Bowman's, anterior stromal, or stromal.

PRE-BOWMAN'S

Manual debridement of the epithelium can always be easily accomplished without difficulty or risk of corneal scarring. As such, manual superficial keratectomy should always be considered initially for pathology confined to the epithelium.

Phototherapeutic ablation of the epithelium with minimal treatment of Bowman's layer may be performed for recurrent epithelial erosions due to epithelial basement membrane abnormalities that fail to respond to more conservative therapy. If the functional needs include correction of a concomitant myopic refractive error, then a photorefractive procedure may be performed in some cases. It should be noted that recurrent epithelial erosions not in the presence of epithelial basement membrane abnormalites are not an FDA-approved indication for the PTK procedure. However, a number of reports have suggested that PTK is effective in some cases of recurrent corneal erosion.[57,58]

BOWMAN'S LAYER

As the depth of the pathology requiring treatment proceeds posteriorly into Bowman's layer, the potential role of phototherapeutic keratectomy acquires increasing favor. It should not, however, lead to automatic consideration of excimer laser ablation, since many disorders of Bowman's layer are easily amenable to manual resection.

If manual superficial keratectomy remains applicable, the same decision-making process as that applied to pre-Bowman's pathology should apply, with the final decision being based on the functional needs of the patient. A classic example is an emmetropic or hyperopic eye with Reis-Buckler's dystrophy or band keratopathy for which manual excision would be the treatment of choice, particularly considering the anticipation of future retreatments for recurrent disease. If the patient is myopic, the initial treatment may be a phototherapeutic or, in selected cases, a photorefractive procedure that, by virtue of removing a portion of the anterior stroma (depending on the degree of myopia), will concomitantly clear the visual axis at the level of Bowman's membrane. Subsequent retreatments can be accomplished by manual means to avoid the induction of hyperopia.

If the lesion is not resectable by manual means, then PTK becomes the only alternative. Examples include a postinfectious scar involving Bowman's layer in the visual axis or smooth climatic droplet keratopathy involving only Bowman's layer, both of which are easily treatable with PTK.[17,22,27,36] If PTK is the only potential treatment, consideration must also be given to the functional needs of the patient before proceeding. For example, an emmetropic patient with a postinfectious scar that is reducing uncorrected and best-corrected visual acuity to 20/30 might perceive a postoperative best-corrected visual acuity of 20/20 a failure if uncorrected visual acuity is reduced significantly due to induced hyperopia. On the other hand, if the visual acuity is reduced to a level that interferes with driving, reading, or other daily activities, the improvement in best-corrected visual acuity may offset the inconvenience of postoperative hyperopia.

Finally, in eyes with combined cataract and corneal opacification (e.g., band keratopathy), concerns about induction of hyperopia become irrelevant if PTK is performed to clear the visual axis as a prelude to subsequent cataract surgery.[17] If cataract surgery is delayed for 3 months, the anterior corneal curvature is sufficiently stable to make intraocular lens calculations that can restore emmetropia.[17]

ANTERIOR STROMAL

With deeper extension into the anterior stroma, manual resection becomes technically more difficult and the risk of postoperative scarring increases. For most anterior stromal disorders, the required amount of excision requires the use of phototherapeutic keratectomy techniques. Skillful PTK (Chapter 3) utilizing a combination of manual debridement of superficial pathology, laser ablation of the epithelium, use of posterior epithelium and masking fluids to smooth the anterior contour, and peripheral blending or "head rocking" to minimize hyperopic shift may produce a functional result that eliminates the need for lamellar or penetrating keratoplasty.[17]

STROMAL

Deep stromal pathology that is adversely affecting visual acuity usually cannot be treated successfully with either manual or PTK. Lamellar or penetrating keratoplasty may be required.

Paracentral Zone

Except in unusual circumstances, disorders affecting the paracentral zone but completely sparing the optical zone should be treated with manual superficial keratectomy when surgical intervention is indicated. In most cases, excision of anterior lesions in the paracentral zone is performed to eliminate ocular surface discomfort, minimize recurrent epithelial erosions, or prevent extension into the visual axis rather than to improve visual acuity. Complete excision of the pathology is usually not required to achieve a surgical cure.

Incomplete surgical excision of a paracentral Salzmann's nodule, for example, may occur with manual techniques, with the potential for residual corneal haze or scarring at the site of the excised nodule. This should have little effect on visual function, but should completely eliminate the foreign body sensation and recurrent epithelial erosions associated with the nodular elevation. PTK, in contrast, may produce more complete excision with a clearer corneal appearance but may alter the contour of Bowman's layer and anterior stroma in normal cornea adjacent to the lesion. If this alteration extends into the visual axis, the induction of irregular astigmatism may result in a decrease in postoperative vision.

Peripheral Zone

As with paracentral pathology, the objective of treatment of superficial corneal pathology in the peripheral zone is usually the management of subjective complaints such as discomfort or optical symptomatology. For most disorders, either manual or phototherapeutic keratectomy will achieve the desired functional result. Because of the distance from the optical zone, however, it is unlikely that unwanted extension of the treatment into the visual axis will occur with PTK if a small treatment zone is used and patient fixation is carefully monitored.

One exception to these principles is with a pterygium, where the indications for surgery may be reduction of irregular astigmatism, ocular motility disturbance, or cosmetic disturbance. Manual excision of the pterygium with a conjunctival autograft[59] or with mitomycin C application[60,61] is preferred to PTK as the primary treatment of choice, although the latter may be used to reduce residual scarring and irregularity following primary excision.

Conclusions

It should be clear from the preceding discussions that PTK is not necessarily the treatment of choice for all anterior corneal pathology. While in many circumstances it represents a significant advance in our ability to excise pathology that was once difficult to remove manually, it does not always guarantee a superior result. In some situations it may produce a less desirable outcome than manual superficial keratectomy. Indeed, the mindset of merely "aiming and shooting" at all pathology that can be reached by the excimer laser will lead to both patient and physician disappointment in many cases.

Corneal surgeons should welcome PTK as a companion to manual superficial keratectomy that affords greater flexibility in tailoring the procedure to the specific clinical situation. Sound clinical evaluation and knowledge of the appropriate indications for both manual superficial keratectomy and PTK will maximize the opportunity for an excellent surgical outcome in a variety of corneal disorders.

References

1. Wagoner MD. Decision making in superficial keratectomy: manual vs. phototherapeutic techniques. Middle Eastern J Ophthalmol 1996;3:181–193.
2. Gangadhar D, Kenyon KR, Wagoner MD. Superficial keratectomy. In Duane T (ed.): Ophthalmology. Vol. 6. Philadelphia: Lippincott, 1994.
3. Starck T, Hersh PS, Kenyon KR. Corneal dysgeneses, dystrophies, and degenerations. In Albert DM, Jakobiec FA (eds.): Principles and Practice of Ophthalmology: Clinical Practice. Vol. 1. Philadelphia: WB Saunders, 1994:13–76.
4. Waring GO III, Rodrigues MM, Laibson PR. Corneal dystrophies. I. Dystrophies of epithelium, Bowman's layer, and stroma. Surv Ophthalmol 1978;23:71–122.

5. Lempert SL, Jenkins MS, Johnson BL, Brown SI. A simple technique for removal of recurring granular dystrophy in corneal grafts. Am J Ophthalmol 1978;86:89–91.

6. Moodaley L, Buckley RJ, Woodward EG. Surgery to improve contact lens wear in keratoconus. CLAO J 1991;17:129–131.

7. Schwartz MF, Taylor HR. Surgical management of Reis-Buckler's corneal dystrophy. Cornea 1985;4:100–107.

8. Wood TO, Walker GG. Treatment of band keratopathy. Am J Ophthalmol 1975;80:553.

9. Wood TO, Fleming JC, Dotson RS, Cotten MS. Treatment of Reis-Buckler's corneal dystrophy by removal of subepithelial fibrous tissue. Am J Ophthalmol 1978;85:360–362.

10. Wood TO. Salzmann's nodular degeneration. Cornea 1990;9:17–22.

11. Buxton JN, Fox ML. Superficial epithelial keratectomy in the treatment of epithelial basement membrane dystrophy. A preliminary report. Arch Ophthalmol 1983;101:392–395.

12. Buckley RJ. Vernal keratopathy and its management. Trans Ophthalmol Soc UK 1981;101:234–238.

13. Kenyon KR, Wagoner MD. Advances in the therapy of recurrent erosion and persistent epithelial defects of the corneal epithelium. Focal Points: Clinical Modules for Ophthalmologists 1991;9.

14. Buxton JN, Constad WH. Superficial epithelial keratectomy in the treatment of epithelial basement membrane dystrophy. Cornea 1987;6:292–297.

15. Breinin GM, DeVoe AG. Chelation of calcium with edathamil calcium-disodium in band keratopathy and corneal calcium affections. Arch Ophthalmol 1954;52:846–851.

16. Bokosky JE, Meyer RF, Sugar A. Surgical treatment of calcific band keratopathy. Ophthalmic Surg 1985;16:645–647.

17. Badr IA, Al-Rajhi AA, Wagoner MD et al. Phototherapeutic keratectomy for climatic droplet keratopathy. J Refract Surg 1996;12:114–122.

18. Cameron JA, Badr IA. Phototherapeutic keratectomy for vernal shield ulcers. J Refract Corneal Surg 1995;11:31–35.

19. Campos M, Nielsen S, Szerenyi K, Gurbus JJ, McDonnell PJ. Clinical follow-up of phototherapeutic keratectomy for treatment of corneal opacities. Ophthalmology 1993;115:433–440.

20. Dausch D, Landesz M, Klein R, Schroder E. Phototherapeutic keratectomy in recurrent corneal epithelial erosion. Refract Corneal Surg 1993;9:419–424.

21. Eiferman RA, Forgey DR, Cook YD. Excimer laser ablation of infectious crystalline keratopathy. Arch Ophthalmol 1992;110:18.

22. Fagerholm P, Fitzsimmons TD, Orndall M et al. Phototherapeutic keratectomy: long term results in 166 eyes. Refract Corneal Surg 1993;9(2 suppl):s76–81.

23. Fitzsimmons TD, Fagerholm P. Superficial keratectomy with the 193 nm excimer laser: a reproducible model of corneal surface irregularities. Acta Ophthalmol 1991;69:641–644.

24. Forster W, Grewe S, Atzler V et al. Phototherapeutic keratectomy in corneal disease. Refract Corneal Surg 1993;9(2 suppl):s585–590.

25. Goldstein M, Loewenstein A, Rosner M et al. Phototherapeutic keratectomy in the treatment of corneal scarring from trachoma. J Refract Surg 1994;10(2 suppl):s290–292.

26. Gottsch JS, Gilbert ML, Goodman DF et al. Excimer laser ablative treatment of microbial keratitis. Ophthalmology 1991;98:146–149.

27. Hahn TW, Sah WJ, Kim JH. Phototherapeutic keratectomy in nine eyes with superficial corneal disease. Refract Corneal Surg 1993:9(2 suppl):s115–118.

28. Hersh PS, Spinak A, Garrana R, Mayers M. Phototherapeutic keratectomy: strategies and results in 12 eyes. Refract Corneal Surg 1993;9(2 suppl):s90–95.

29. John ME, Van der Kaff MA, Noblitt RL, Boleyn KL. Excimer laser phototherapeutic keratectomy for treatment of recurrent corneal erosion. J Refract Surg 1994;20:179–181.

30. Lohmann CP, Sachs H, Marshall J, Gabel VP. Excimer laser phototherapeutic keratectomy for recurrent erosions: a clinical study. Ophthalmic Surg Lasers 1996;27:768–772.

31. John ME, Matines E, Cvintal T, Ballew C. Excimer laser photoablation of primary familial amyloidosis of the cornea. Refract Corneal Surg 1993;9(2 suppl):s138–141.

32. Lawless MA, Cohen P, Rogers C. Phototherapeutic keratectomy for Reis-Buckler's dystrophy. Refract Corneal Surg 1993;9(2 suppl):s96–98.

33. L'Esperance FA, Warner JW, Telfair WB et al. Excimer laser instrumentation and technique for human corneal surgery. Arch Ophthalmol 1989;107:131–139.

34. McDonnell PJ, Sieler T. Phototherapeutic keratectomy with excimer laser for Reis-Buckler's corneal dystrophy. Refract Corneal Surg 1992;8:306–310.

35. Moodaley L, Liu C, Woodward EG, O'Brart D, Muir MK, Buckley R. Excimer laser superficial keratectomy or proud nebulae in keratoconus. Br J Ophthalmol 1994;78:454–457.
36. O'Brart DS, Gartry DS, Lohmann CP, Patmore AL, Muir MGK, Marshall J. Treatment of band keratopathy by excimer laser phototherapeutic keratectomy: surgical techniques and long term follow up. Br J Ophthalmol 1993;77:702–708.
37. Rapuano CJ, Laibson PR. Excimer laser phototherapeutic keratectomy. CLAO J 1993;19:235–240.
38. Rogers C, Cohen P, Lawless M. Phototherapeutic keratectomy for Reis-Buckler's corneal dystrophy. Aust NZ J Ophthalmol 1993;21:247–250.
39. Sedaravec O, Darrell RW, Krieger RR, Trokel SL. Excimer laser therapy for experimental *Candida* keratitis. Am J Ophthalmol 1985;99:534–538.
40. Sher NA, Bowers RA, Zabel RW et al. Clinical use of 193 nm excimer laser in the treatment of corneal scars. Arch Ophthalmol 1991;109:491–498.
41. Stark WJ, Chamon W, Kamp MT, Engler CL, Renes EV, Gottsch JD. Clinical follow-up of 193-nm ArF excimer laser photokeratectomy. Ophthalmology 1992;99:805–812.
42. Steinert RF, Puliafito CA. Excimer laser phototherapeutic keratectomy for a corneal nodule. Refract Corneal Surg 1990;6:352.
43. Talamo JH, Steinert RF, Puliafito CA. Clinical strategies for excimer laser therapeutic keratectomy. Refract Corneal Surg 1992;8:319–324.
44. Steinert RF. Therapeutic keratectomy: corneal smoothing. In Thompson FB, McDonnell PJ (eds.): Excimer Laser Surgery. Tokyo: Igaku-Shoin, 1993:121–130.
45. Thompson V, Durrie DS, Cavanaugh TB. Philosophy and technique for excimer laser phototherapeutic keratectomy. Ophthalmology 1993;9(2 suppl):s81–85.
46. Trokel SL, Srinivasan R, Braren B. Excimer laser surgery of the cornea. Am J Ophthalmol 1983;96:710–715.
47. Fountain TR, de la Cruz Z, Green WR et al. Reassembly of corneal epithelial adhesion structures after excimer laser keratectomy in humans. Arch Ophthalmol 1994;112:967–972.
48. Kornmehl EW, Steinert RF, Puliafito CA. A comparative study of masking fluids for excimer laser phototherapeutic keratectomy. Arch Ophthalmol 1991;109:860–863.
49. Seiler T, Bende T, Wollensak J. Ablation rate of human corneal epithelium and Bowman's layer with the excimer laser (193 nm). Refract Corneal Surg 1990;6:99–102.
50. McDonnell JM, Garbus JJ, McDonnell PJ. Unsuccessful excimer laser phototherapeutic keratectomy. Clinicopathologic correlation. Arch Ophthalmol 1992;110:977–979.
51. Hersh PS, Jordan AJ, Mayers M. Corneal graft rejection episode after excimer laser phototherapeutic keratectomy. Arch Ophthalmol 1993;11:735–736.
52. Vrabec MP, Anderson JA, Rock ME et al. Electron microscopic findings in a cornea with recurrence of herpes simplex keratitis after excimer laser phototherapeutic keratectomy. CLAO J 1994;20:41–44.
53. Wu WC, Stark WJ, Green WR. Corneal wound healing after 193-nm excimer laser kratectomy. Arch Ophthalmol 1991;10:1426–1432.
54. Binder PS, Anderson JA, Rock ME, Vrabec MP. Human excimer laser keratectomy. Clinical and histopathologic correlations. Ophthalmology 1994;101:979–989.
55. Al-Rajhi A, Wagoner MD, Badr IA, Al-Saif A, Mahmood M. Infectious keratitis following phototherapeutic keratectomy. J Refract Surg 1996;12:123–127.
56. Waring GO III. FDA panel recommends conditional approval of excimer laser phototherapeutic keratectomy (PTK). J Refract Surg 1994;10:77–78.
57. John ME, Van Der Karr MA, Noblitt RL, Boleyn KL. Excimer laser phototherapeutic keratectomy for the treatment of recurrent corneal erosion. J Cataract Refract Surg. 1994;20:179–81.
58. Dausch D, Landesz M, Klein R, Schroder E. Phototherapeutic keratectomy in recurrent epithelial erosion.
59. Kenyon KR, Wagoner MD, Hettinger ME. Conjunctival autograft transplantation for advanced and recurrent pterygium. Ophthalmology 1985;92:1461–1470.
60. Wagoner MD, Sieck EA. Short term adjunctive mitomycin-C therapy following pterygium excision. Middle Eastern J Ophthalmol 1995;3:6–10.
61. Singh G, Wilson MR, Foster CS. Mitomycin-C eye drops as treatment of pterygium. Ophthalmology 1988;95:813–821.

3

Techniques of Excimer Laser Phototherapeutic Keratectomy

The phototherapeutic keratectomy procedure in general subsumes a variety of specific surgical strategies. Proper recognition of indications and appropriate case selection will suggest which of a variety of specific surgical techniques to undertake (Table 3–1). The specific surgical strategy will vary significantly with different corneal disorders as indicated by the therapeutic decision-making algorithm (see Chapter 2). Clinical goals and functional objectives of the procedure may, likewise, vary depending on the patient's symptomatology. In addition, the side effects and complications of the various PTK surgical strategies may differ from both PRK and those of manual superficial keratectomy and thus must be anticipated when choosing treatment of superficial corneal disease.

This chapter details each of the specific surgical strategies employed in manual and laser-assisted superficial keratectomy for the optimum treatment of the diverse group of superficial corneal pathologies.

Preoperative Preparation

In general, superficial keratectomy with or without the laser should be performed on a quiet eye. Possible confounding problems such as blepharitis and active infection should be controlled before proceeding with surgery. Eyes with active herpetic keratitis should be avoided. Ocular inflammation should be controlled (see Chapter 5).

Once it has been decided that the laser will be used, it must first be tested. As discussed in Chapter 1, appropriate laser energy and beam homogeneity

Table 3–1   Corneal Disorders and Potential Surgical Strategy

General large area PTK
  Corneal dystrophies
    Reis-Buckler's dystrophy
    Lattice dystrophy
    Granular dystrophy
    Schneider's crystalline dystrophy
    Epithelial basement membrane dystrophy
    Meesman's dystrophy
  Corneal degenerations
    Climatic droplet keratopathy
    Amyloid degeneration
    Diffuse Salzmann's degeneration
  Corneal irregularities
    Associated with dystrophies and degenerations
    Irregular astigmatism following penetrating keratoplasty
    Following pterygium removal
Combined manual superficial keratectomy and PTK
    Calcific band keratopathy
    Focal climatic droplet keratopathy
    Pterygium
    Focal nodules
    Keratoconus apical nodules
Focal smoothing
    Salzmann's nodular degeneration
    Apical nodules in keratoconus
    Focal irregularities following surgery or infection
Superficial scar removal
    Herpetic keratitis scars
    Following corneal infections
    Traumatic scars
Epithelial adherence disorders
    Epithelial basement membrane dystrophy
    Contact lens keratopathy
    Selected cases of epithelial dysadherence syndromes

should be ensured before any laser treatment. In some cases, to facilitate centration of the procedure, the operative eye may receive pilocarpine 1% to constrict the pupil to improve visualization when aiming the laser. Most procedures are done using only topical anesthetic drops. To ensure a proper radiant energy density on the cornea, the patient's eye is brought to the proper vertical plane.

Training sessions may be performed in some cases to familiarize the patient with the laser procedure. The application of methylcellulose 1% to the cornea before ablation will block the incoming laser beam and allow the patient to become accustomed to the sensations of laser application. In some cases when the epithelium will be manually removed before PTK, laser first may be applied to the epithelium using approximately 25 pulses to better demonstrate the sensations of the treatment to the patient.

Techniques

Manual Superficial Keratectomy

Instrumentation for superficial keratectomy consists of dry cellulose sponges, fine-toothed forceps (e.g., 0.12 mm) or jeweler's forceps, and a rounded spatula-type microsurgical blade. Epithelium over the involved area is removed by wiping with cellulose sponges or gentle scraping with the blade, avoiding sharp dissection or nicking of the underlying Bowman's layer and stroma (Fig. 3–1). Care is taken to leave peripheral corneal and limbal epithelium intact in order to provide a reservoir of cells for subsequent epithelialization.[1]

A cleavage plane is identified between abnormal tissue and Bowman's layer or stroma using dry cellulose sponges, the microsurgical blade, or a blunt spatula to raise a tissue edge. To facilitate visualization and manipulation of the abnormal tissue, the corneal surface is kept dry. Traction may be applied with forceps to strip the abnormal material along its natural cleavage plane, while the tip of a dry cellulose sponge may be used as an attraumatic dissecting instrument (Fig. 3–2). In the case of strong adherence, the blade may be carefully used to lyse adhesions or to scrape residual abnormal tissue. Caution should always be taken to remain in the cleavage plane, thus avoiding damage to Bowman's membrane that may evoke further corneal scarring and irregularity. After stripping, the corneal surface may be further smoothed by scrubbing with cellulose sponges or gentle scraping with the back edge of the blade.

In the case of band keratopathy, EDTA (0.35%) may be used to chelate residual intrastromal calcium deposits.

CASE 1

History and preoperative evaluation. A 76-year-old Vietnamese male complained of poor vision in both eyes. On examination his best corrected visual acuity was counts fingers (CF) at 8 feet in the right eye and 20/200 in the left eye. On slit-lamp examination there was a visually significant pterygium extending into the paracentral cornea from the nasal quadrant in both eyes and from the temporal quadrant of the right eye. There were visually significant cataracts bilaterally. Fundoscopic examination was normal in both eyes. On keratometry the mires were very irregular, with at least 8 diopters of nasal flattening in both eyes.

Over the next 16 months he underwent bilateral cataract extraction, YAG capsulotomy, and pterygium excision. In April 1992, the uncorrected visual acuity in the right eye was 20/200, improving to 20/60 with plano $-3.75 \times$ 85. In the left eye the uncorrected visual acuity was 20/100, improving to 20/50 with $+0.25 -3.75 \times 105$. Keratometry showed mild nasal flattening and irregularity in both eyes with mild irregular astigmatism in the visual

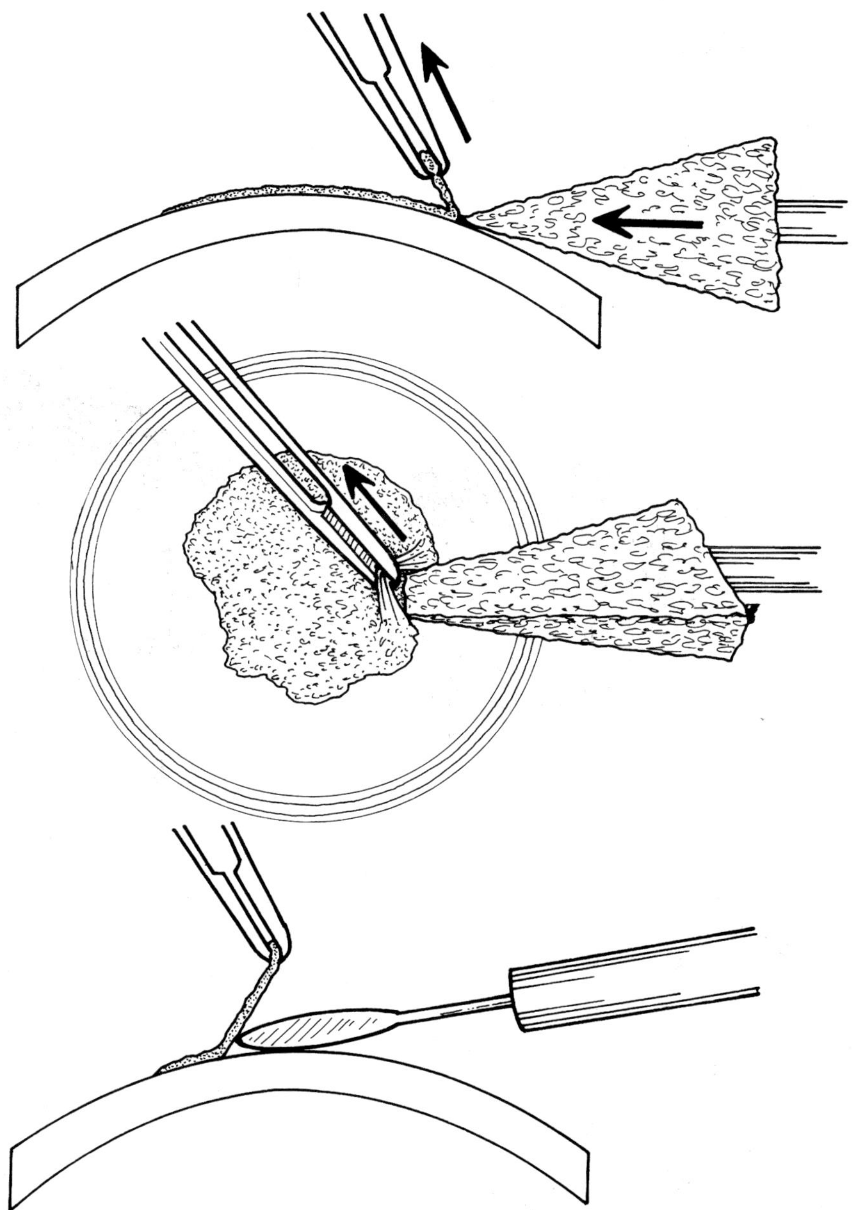

Figure 3–1.   Technique of superficial keratectomy. A dry cellulose sponge is used to identify a cleavage plane beneath the abnormal tissue. The tissue is peeled along the plane using tissue forceps and blunt dissection. A spatula-type blade may be used to free firmly adherent tissue, keeping the blade parallel to the cornea to avoid damage to underlying stroma.

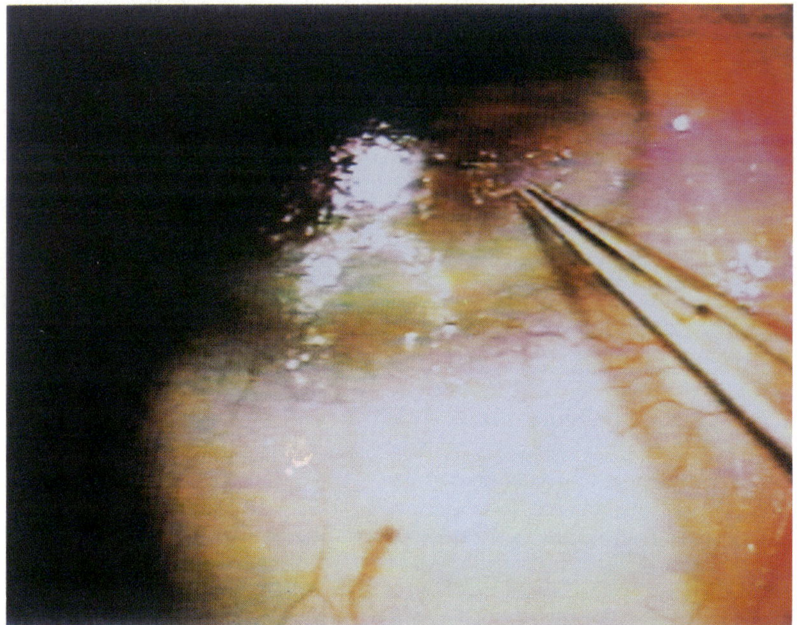

A

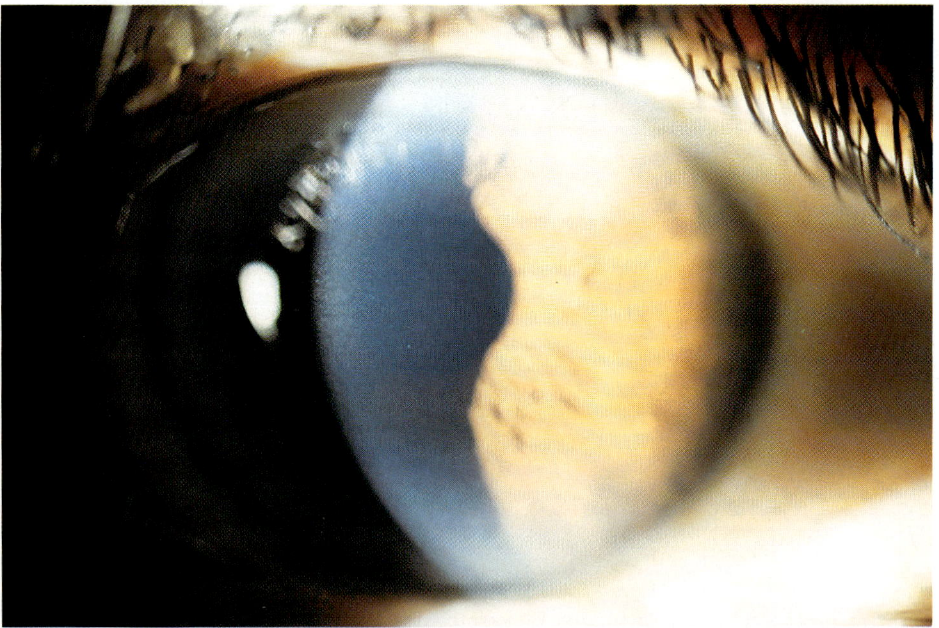

B

Figure 3–2.   This 70-year-old woman presented with a complaint of ocular surface discomfort secondary to a Salzmann's nodule. Best corrected vision was 20/40^{-1}. **(A)** Intraoperative photograph demonstrates a peeling and stripping technique with 0.12 mm forceps and dry cellulose sponges. The nodule is stripped from underlying stroma along a lamellar cleavage plane. **(B)** One month postoperatively, the cornea is clear.

axis. The visual axis in the right eye had residual diffuse anterior stromal scarring without epithelial irregularity.

Over the next 10 months, he complained of gradually painless decreased vision in his right eye. On examination, his best-corrected visual acuity had deteriorated to CF at 8 feet. On slit-lamp examination, the previously documented anterior stromal haze in the visual axis was unchanged, but a subepithelial, Salzmann's-like nodule had developed superior temporally, with extension of the proximal edge to within 1 mm of the visual axis (Fig. 3–3). Computerized corneal topography showed dramatic steeping (60–70 diopters) in the superior temporal quadrant of the 3 mm optical zone with a commensurate flattening (35–40 diopters) in the inferior nasal quadrant. The visual center was markedly steepened (62.4 diopters) (Fig. 3–4).

Algorithmic analysis.

Horizontal assessment. The pathology is in the central optical zone (green color code), allowing consideration of possible phototherapeutic keratectomy, pending further analysis of other parameters.

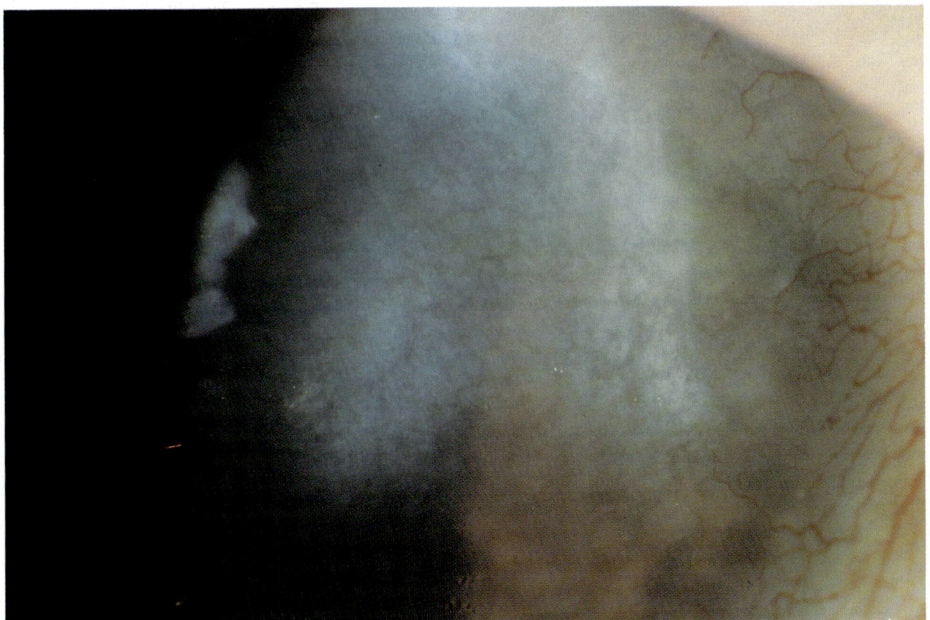

Figure 3–3.   Case 1. Note a paracentral Salzmann's-like nodule superior temporal to the visual axis. Mild anterior stromal scarring is present in the visual axis. (Reproduced with permission from Wagoner and Waller.[24])

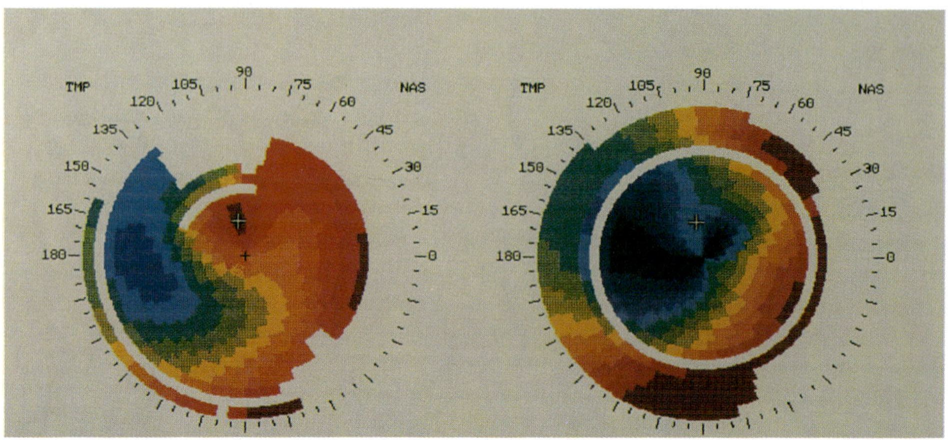

Figure 3–4.   Case 1. Computerized corneal topography preoperatively shows **(Left)** marked steeping (60–70 diopters) in the superior temporal quadrant, extending into the visual axis, with a commensurate flattening of the inferior nasal quadrant (less than 40 diopters). At the site of the cursor (+), the corneal steepness is 62.4 diopters. **(Right)** After manual superficial keratectomy, there is elimination of the superior temporal steepening, visual axis steepening, inferior nasal flattening, and elimination of the 20–25 diopter curvature disparity between the superior temporal and inferior nasal quadrants. At the site of the cursor (+), the corneal steepness is 44.6 diopters, indicating overall corneal flattening of 17.8 diopters. (Reproduced with permission from Wagoner and Waller.[24])

PATTERN OF PATHOLOGY.   In this case, there is nodular pathology adjacent to the optical center, as well as diffuse anterior stromal pathology in the optical center.

Based on the history of initial good visual acuity in the presence of the diffuse anterior stromal haze, the deterioration of the visual acuity concomitantly with the development of the Salzmann's-like nodule, and the confirmatory computerized corneal topography of marked irregular astigmatism, it is clear that the approach to therapy is removal of the corneal nodule. According to the second level of the algorithm, excision of an isolated nodule in the optical zone should be performed by manual keratectomy (red color code) unless there are strong mitigating circumstances requiring phototherapeutic ablation.

Surgical therapy and outcome.   Manual superficial keratectomy was performed with topical anesthesia, with complete excision of the paracentral nodule. Following removal of his surgical dressing on the first postoperative day, the visual acuity was dramatically improved to 20/40 without correction. Repeat corneal topography 1 week later showed flattening of the central cornea by nearly 18 diopters, as well as complete elimination of the irregular astigmatism in the superior temporal and inferior nasal quadrants (Fig. 3–4).

CASE 2

History and preoperative evaluation.   A 44-year-old white female with long-standing keratoconus in both eyes had undergone penetrating keratoplasty in the right eye in 1971 and had been managed with hard contact lens wear in both eyes since that time for visual rehabilitation.

In 1972, the uncorrected visual acuity in the right eye was 20/80, improving to 20/20 with either a spectacle correction of $+1.00 -4.75 \times 147$ or a hard contact lens. Keratometry readings were 39.00×10 and 46.50×95. Her contact lens wear and visual acuity remained stable for the next 13 years.

Between 1985 and 1992, she had progressive contact lens difficulties in the right eye, requiring frequent refitting. During this period, slowly progressive subepithelial fibrous tissue was documented in the graft on serial examinations. Uncorrected visual acuity and spectacle-corrected acuity had both deteriorated to CF at 5 feet, although hard contact lens acuity was 20/30. Keratometry showed central corneal steepening with 50.50×180 and 53.00×90. Unfortunately, the best possible contact lens fit did not result in sufficient comfort or stability to permit lens wear. Slit-lamp examination revealed subepithelial fibrous pannus extending into the central portion of the graft from the nasal quadrant with slight superior extension (Fig. 3–5). A rigid contact lens was very unstable and was easily extruded from the eye with firm blink. Computerized corneal topography showed very irregular astigmatism with marked steepening in the nasal and superior quadrant of the graft (>55 diopters) with the steepest area (59.4 diopters) just superior to the optical center (Fig. 3–6). The area of keratometric steepening corresponded to the distribution of subepithelial fibrous pannus.

Algorithmic Analysis

HORIZONTAL ASSESSMENT.   The pathology is in the central optical zone (green color code), allowing consideration of possible phototherapeutic keratectomy, pending further analysis of other parameters.

PATTERN OF PATHOLOGY.   In this case, there is segmental pathology adjacent to the optical center. Two possible etiologies of the decreased visual acuity are irregular astigmatism as demonstrated by computerized corneal topography, as well clouding of the visual axis due to the haze in the optical zone. The hard contact lens acuity of 20/30 suggests that most of the patient's complaints are due to the irregular astigmatism. According to the second level of the algorithm, excision of segmental pathology in the optical zone should be performed by manual keratectomy (red color code) unless there are strong mitigating circumstances requiring phototherapeutic ablation. The

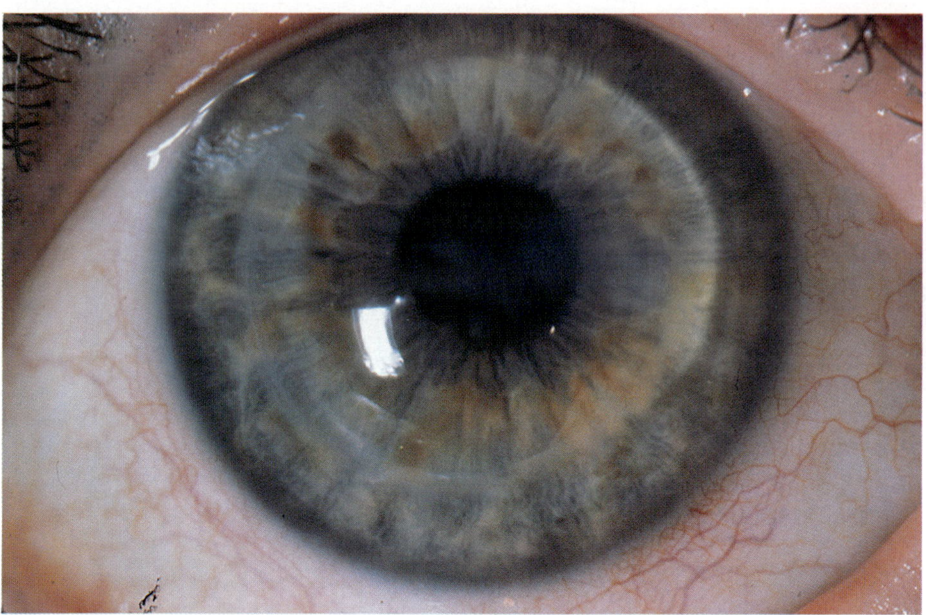

Figure 3–5.   Case 2. Note a subepithelial fibrous plaque extending across the nasal portion of the corneal graft with extension into the visual axis and superior quadrant. (Reproduced with permission from Wagoner and Waller.[24])

only such mitigating circumstance would be related to concerns that complete clearing of Bowman's membrane is required to achieve a satisfactory acuity. If this were the case, the proper treatment would still be manual excision of the pathology followed by minimal polishing of Bowman's membrane with the excimer laser using a well-centered ablation of the central optical zone.

Surgical therapy and outcome.   Manual superficial keratectomy was performed with topical anesthesia. The subepithelial fibrous tissue was easily peeled from normal underlying cornea. One month postoperatively, the uncorrected visual acuity had improved to 20/100 in the right eye. Visual acuity was 20/40 with a +1.00 −2.25 × 25, while hard contact lens acuity was 20/20. It was possible to fit a stable, comfortable hard contact lens. Slit-lamp examination showed nearly complete removal of the subepithelial pannus with faint nebular scarring of Bowman's membrane (Fig. 3–7). Computerized corneal topography showed a dramatic reduction in the steepest area of the paracentral cornea, overall reduction in central corneal steepness, and much less irregular astigmatism (Fig. 3–6).

General Large Area PTK

This technique is used for diffuse superficial corneal opacities and irregularities such as Reis-Buckler's, lattice, and other corneal dystrophies; general-

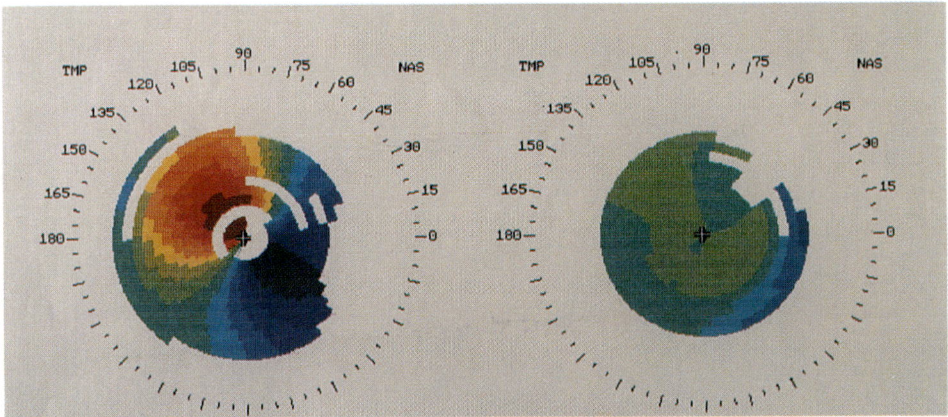

Figure 3–6.   Case 2. Computerized corneal topography preoperatively shows **(Left)** a marked central, superior, and nasal corneal steepening with irregular astigmatism. At the site of the cursor (+), the corneal steepness is 59.4 diopters. **(Right)** Following manual superficial keratectomy, there is a marked reduction in irregular astigmatism. At the site of the cursor (+) the corneal steepness is 47.5 diopters, indicating an overall corneal flattening of 11.9 diopters. (Reproduced with permission from Wagoner and Waller.[24])

ized superficial keratopathies; and other extensive corneal surface irregularities (Fig. 3–8).

If the epithelial surface is irregular, it is carefully removed using dry cellulose sponges and the back of a spatula-type blade avoiding damage to underlying stroma. Care is taken to leave peripheral corneal and limbal epithelium intact as in the manual superficial keratectomy procedure. In contrast, if the corneal epithelial surface appears to be smoothing the surface of a more irregular underlying stroma, it may be left in place and removed with the laser. In this way, the epithelium will mask the irregularities of the subjacent stroma, acting as a biological "spackle," and leaving a smoother postoperative surface.

For general large area PTK, a wide diameter spot size (e.g. 5–6 mm) is generally selected. It is important to note that, in general, the excimer laser will remove an equivalent amount of tissue (approximately 0.25 μm/pulse) over the entire area upon which it impinges. Although opacities will be removed, irregularities of the surface will be maintained because tissue is removed parallel to the surface. Therefore, of particular importance for the PTK procedure, a nonsmooth corneal surface must be "spackled" with methycellulose 1% to fill in irregularities, thereby smoothing the surface to be ablated (Fig. 3–9).[2–4] The viscosity of methylcellulose 1% generally is appropriate to fill in the "valleys" of an irregular surface while leaving the "peaks" exposed. This allows the surface to be smoothed with the laser while opac-

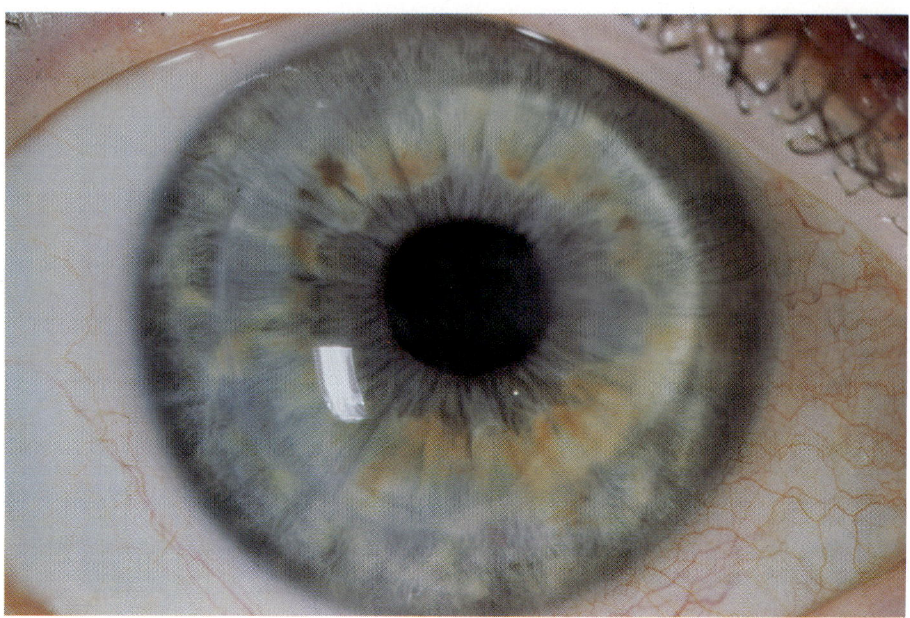

Figure 3–7.   Case 2. Postoperatively, while the elevated portion of the subepithelial fibrous plaque has been "stripped" by manual superficial keratectomy, there is still a faint, visually insignificant nebular scar present at the level of Bowman's membrane. (Reproduced with permission from Wagoner and Waller.[24])

ities are removed. Concentrations of methylcellulose less than 1% may flow too freely; higher concentrations tend to completely mask the incoming beam. The thickness of the methylcellulose layer should be enough to smooth the valleys of the corneal surface, but not so much as to completely block the incoming laser beam. For example, one case of Reis-Buckler's dystrophy required 1,095 pulses and was done early in the authors' experience. Her second eye, completed approximately 6 months later, required approximately 600 pulses. Since the postoperative pachymetry reading was similar after both procedures, this decreased laser treatment likely reflected an improvement in surgical technique with more appropriate methylcellulose application in the second eye. An overly muted sound of the laser–tissue interaction may signal to the surgeon that too much methylcellulose has been applied. Collagen gels and other molding compounds hold promise for future use in the PTK procedure to provide an even smoother postoperative corneal surface.[3]

After focusing the laser and centering the eye,[5] the laser procedure is begun. With the patient gazing at the laser's fixation light, the footpedal is depressed and lasing proceeds as the eye is rotated by gently moving the patient's head (Fig. 3–8). This is in contrast to the "point-and-shoot" tech-

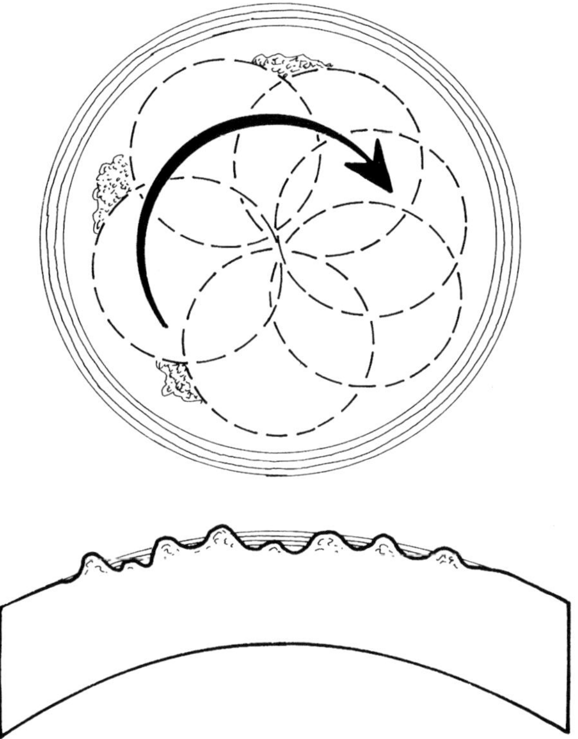

Figure 3–8.   Technique of general large area PTK. Schematic showing methylcellulose filling in valleys of an irregular corneal surface. Annular movement of eye under laser beam smooths and clears a large surface area of the cornea.

nique used in PRK; in PTK, the annular eye motion blends the edge of the ablation zone, avoiding the creation of a stromal crater with a sharp perpendicular edge with its consequent distortion of corneal surface topography. This "polishing" technique with the use of smoothing agents also mitigates hyperopic refractive shifts from the procedure (see Chapter 6).[6]

The surgeon must be aware of the rate and pattern of tissue ablation during PTK. Sensory feedback can serve as a guide. During the procedure, a blue fluorescence signals that epithelium is being ablated.[7] This fluorescence disappears upon reaching the corneal stroma because of its lower water content. To best visualize this epithelial fluorescence, room lights should be turned off and the illumination on the laser turned down. Methylcellulose, in contrast, tends to whiten and bubble upon ablation, and the normal loud snapping sound of the laser–tissue interaction is muffled, indicating partial masking of the incoming beam. If the sound is substantially muffled, removal of tissue will be minimal. An intermediate sound usually indicates satisfactory masking of tissue valleys while peaks remain exposed to laser ablation.

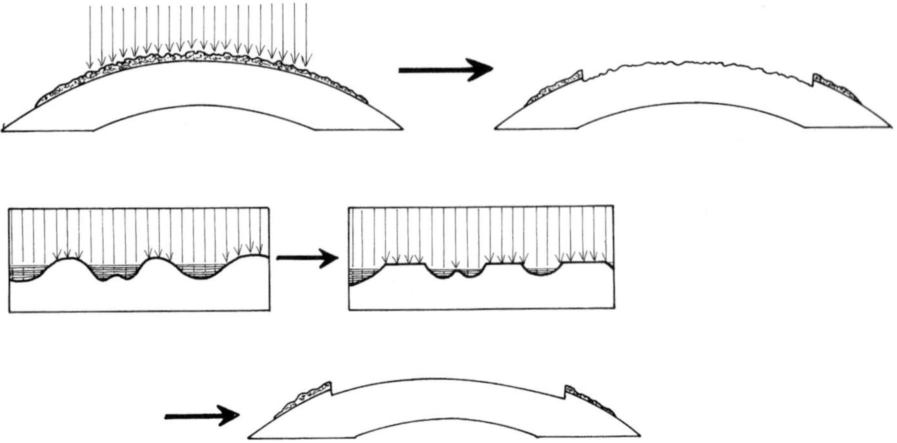

Figure 3–9.   Schematic depicting an irregular corneal surface before **(Upper left)** and after **(Upper right)** excimer laser ablation. Note how the corneal surface pattern is preserved although the corneal substance is thinned. Using a masking compound to protect the "valleys" of the corneal surface by absorbing the incoming laser energy **(Middle left)** will allow smoothing of the surface as the "peaks" of the irregular surface are removed by photoablation **(Middle right)** leaving a smooth corneal surface **(Bottom)**.

The procedure is interrupted at relative frequent intervals, and the patient is examined frequently at the slit lamp to monitor the progress of the procedure and to determine areas to be treated further. Having a slit lamp near the laser room is helpful. Additional methylcellulose is applied as necessary to smooth the surface as the procedure proceeds. Adequately treated areas may be protected from further laser ablation by focally applying a thick layer of methylcellulose 1% or 2.5%. A relatively high concentration (1% or 2.5%) is preferred since thinner solutions tend to flow from the intended area (Fig. 3–10). Moreover, the beam diameter may be changed as necessary to touch-up remaining areas of pathology and to avoid unintended ablation of areas adequately treated.

To decrease irregular astigmatism, relatively more treatment may be applied to steep areas as evidenced by the videokeratography map. In particular, investigators have suggested focal applications of the laser in steep areas of the corneal topography map to reduce irregular astigmatism. By using the equation, $t = s^2D/3$, where t = center thickness in microns, s = diameter of the ablation, and D = correction in diopters, they calculate the depth of zones of relative steepening as determined by a computer-assisted videokeratography map.[9] Using a nominal ablation rate of 0.25 μm for each excimer laser pulse, an ablation pattern is delivered in an attempt to decrease the irregular astigmatism (Fig. 3–11). Such a technique must be planned with caution, however, and videokeratography maps must be analyzed properly.

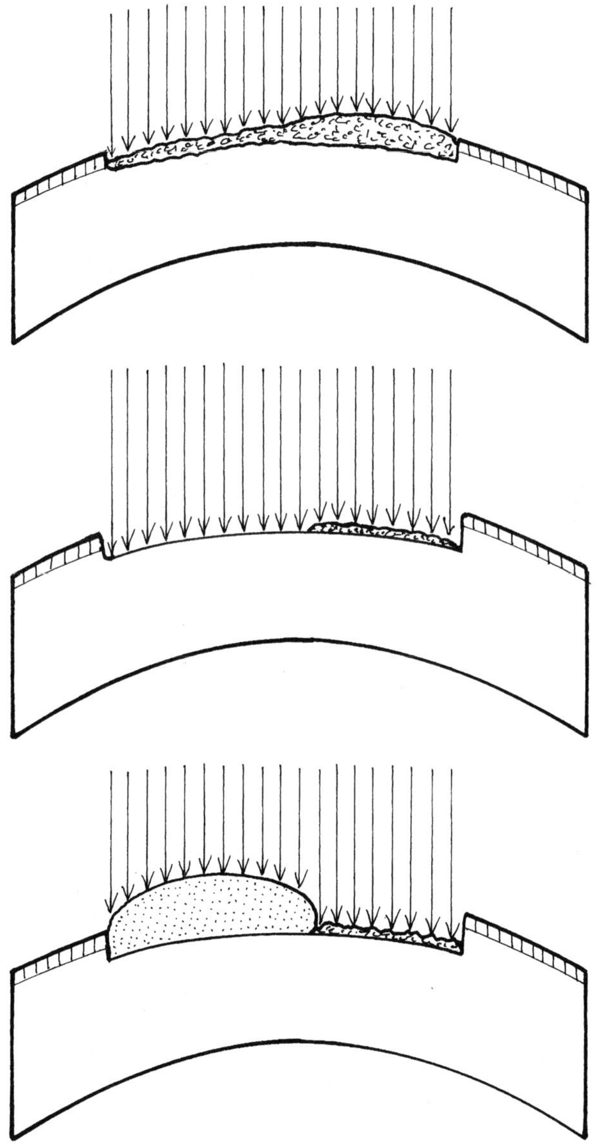

Figure 3–10.   The patient is examined at the slit lamp, and adequately treated areas are protected from further laser ablation by focal application of a relatively viscous masking agent.

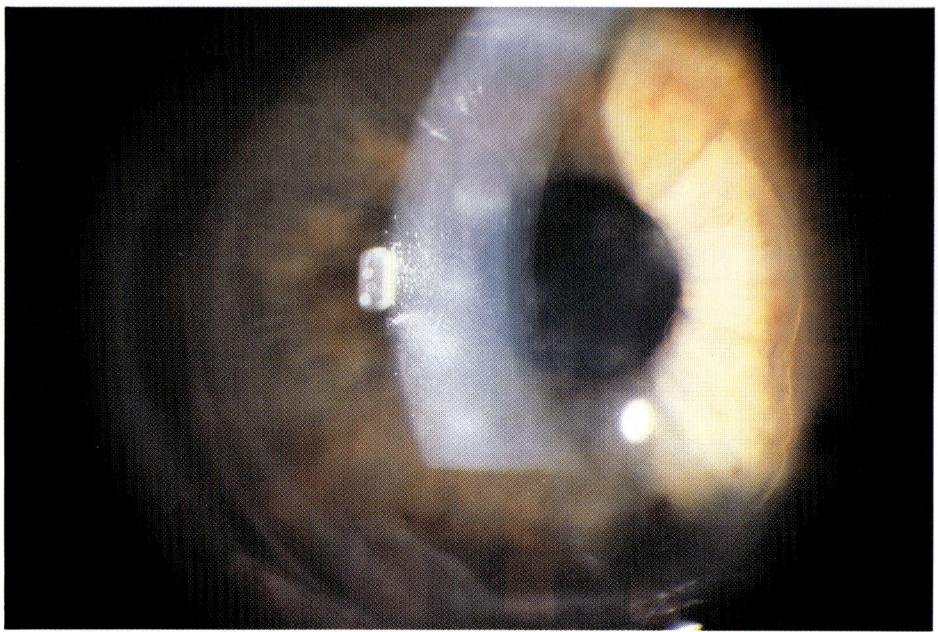

Figure 3–11.   Case 3. **(A)** A 54-year-old woman had spectacle corrected visual acuity of 20/200 following penetrating keratoplasty, secondary to subepithelial scarring and irregular astigmatism. *(Continued on following page)*

The surgeon must determine whether an area of steep curvature is elevated or depressed. In the latter case, further removal of tissue by laser ablation may exacerbate, rather than improve, irregular astigmatism.[25]

Furthermore, some investigators advocate placing a midperipheral annulus of treatment using a small beam diameter (e.g., 2 mm) to steepen the overall macroscopic corneal contour, thus minimizing hyperopic shifts induced by the procedure (Fig. 3–12).[10,11] Such an intervention may be useful if the border of the ablation zone and peripheral cornea appears abrupt. In this technique, the smaller beam is used to meticulously smooth and blend the junction of the treated and nontreated cornea.

At the conclusion of the treatment, the cornea typically has a ground-glass appearance. Although the cornea may not be completely cleared, treatment should be minimized, since relatively large amounts of tissue might be removed with this technique with consequent refractive shifts and topographic irregularities.[12] After epithelial healing, corneal luster is regained and visual acuity may be markedly improved despite residual opacities.

CASE 4

History and preoperative evaluation.   A 31-year-old woman with Reis-Buckler's dystrophy was seen with a best-corrected visual acuity of 20/200 and uncorrected visual acuity of 20/400 with a refraction of −6.50 diopters (Fig. 3–13).

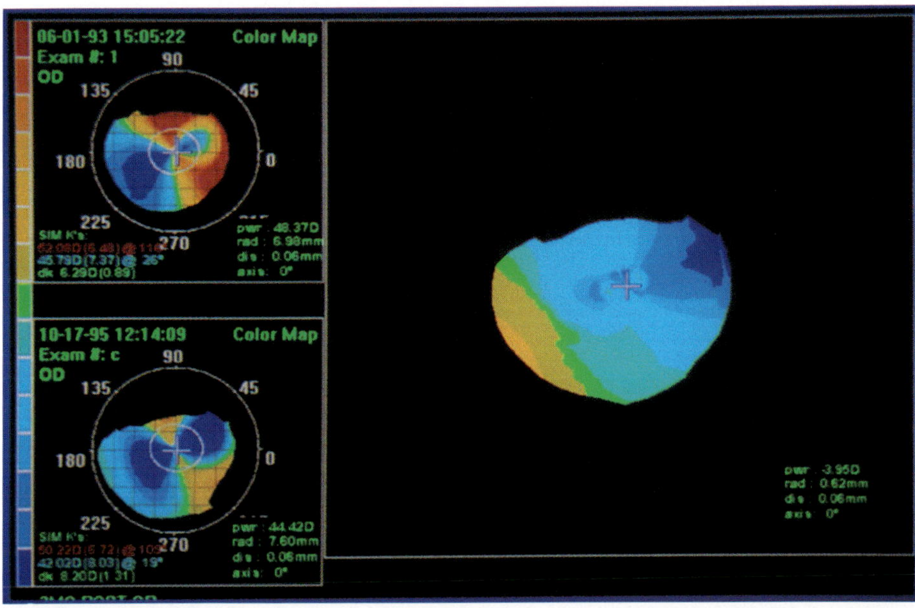

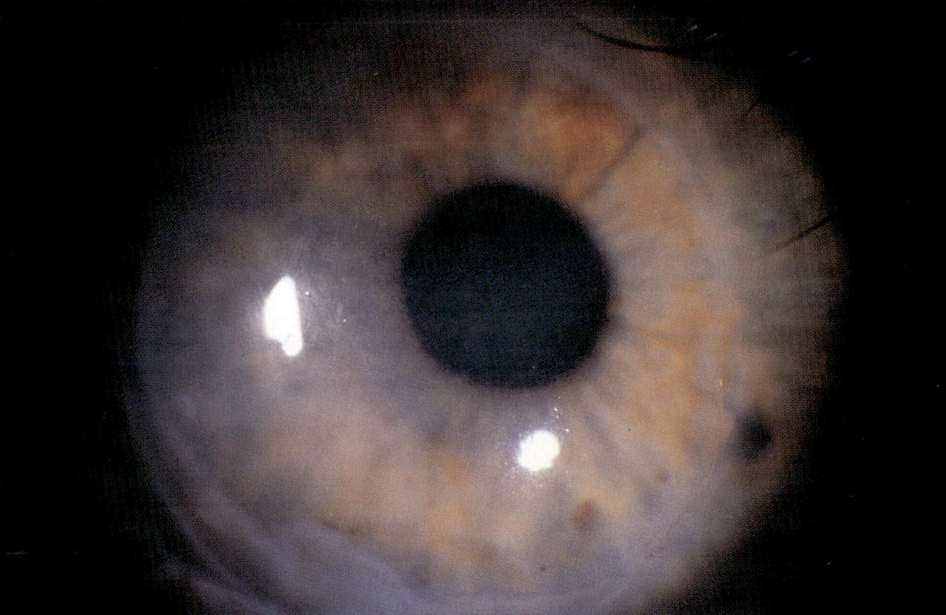

Figure 3–11 (B, top left).   The preoperative videokeratography map shows irregular astigmatism with corneal steepening at 12 o'clock and 4 o'clock. Following general large area PTK, the beam diameter was decreased to 4 mm and additional treatment was applied to the steep (red) areas. **(B, bottom left)** The postoperative topography map shows improvement in the irregular astigmatism. **(B, right)** The differential topography map shows flattening of the previously steep areas. **(C)** Three months postoperatively, the cornea is cleared with improvement in irregular astigmatism and improved spectacle corrected visual acuity to 20/60.

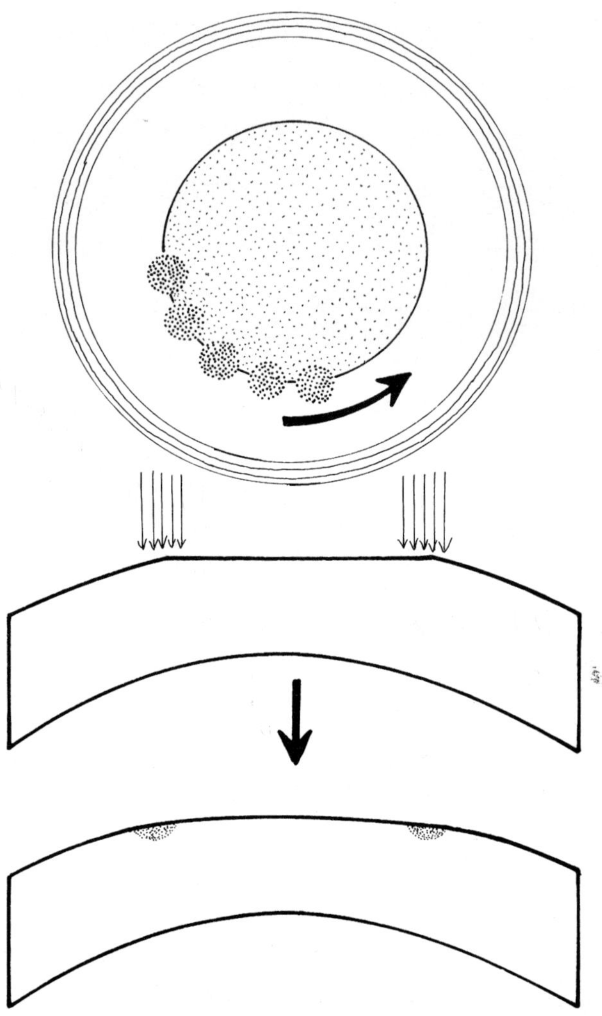

Figure 3–12.   After central corneal treatment, a midperipheral annulus of treatment using a small beam diameter is placed to blend the edges and minimize corneal flattening by steepening the macroscopic corneal contour.

Algorithmic analysis.

HORIZONTAL ASSESSMENT AND PATTERN.   The pathology is in the central optical zone (green color code) and extends to the periphery encompassing the entire cornea.

VERTICAL ASSESSMENT.   On slit-lamp examination, the pathologic process appears to encompass Bowman's layer and the superficial stroma. The epithelium appears smooth.

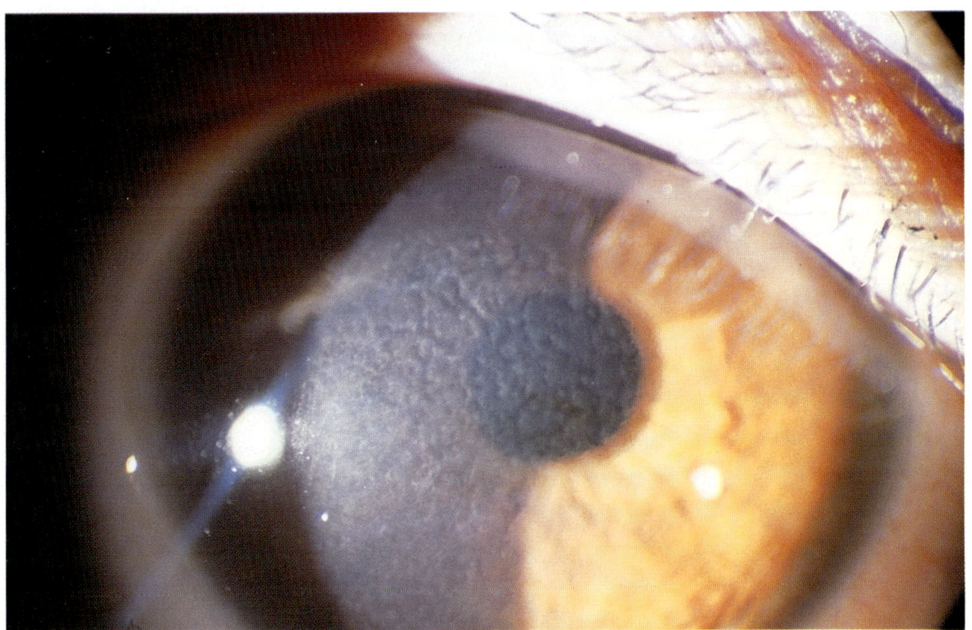

Figure 3–13.   Case 4. **(A)** Preoperative appearance of a 31-year-old woman with Reis-Buckler's dystrophy and best-corrected visual acuity of 20/200 with a refraction of −6.50. *(Continued on following page)*

Surgical therapy and outcome.   The goal of the procedure in this case is to improve visual acuity. General large area PTK using the polishing technique and masking methylcellulose 1% was performed using 1,065 pulses of the laser and a 6.0 mm beam diameter. Immediately following surgery, some dystrophic material remained, and the cornea demonstrated a ground-glass appearance on slit-lamp examination. Six months postoperatively, the cornea was clear with restoration of best-corrected spectacle visual acuity to 20/30 with a refraction of −2.50. A similar procedure was performed on the patient's other eye with similar results. Results have been stable for 3 years postoperatively.

CASE 5

History and preoperative evaluation.   A 41-year-old woman with lattice corneal dystrophy had previously undergone successful penetrating keratoplasty (Fig. 3–14). Six years later, best-corrected visual acuity in the left eye had decreased from 20/25 to 20/80 because of recurrent lattice in the graft. The patient also complained of ocular surface discomfort. Lattice deposits were seen beneath the epithelium and in the superficial corneal stroma with a markedly irregular corneal surface.

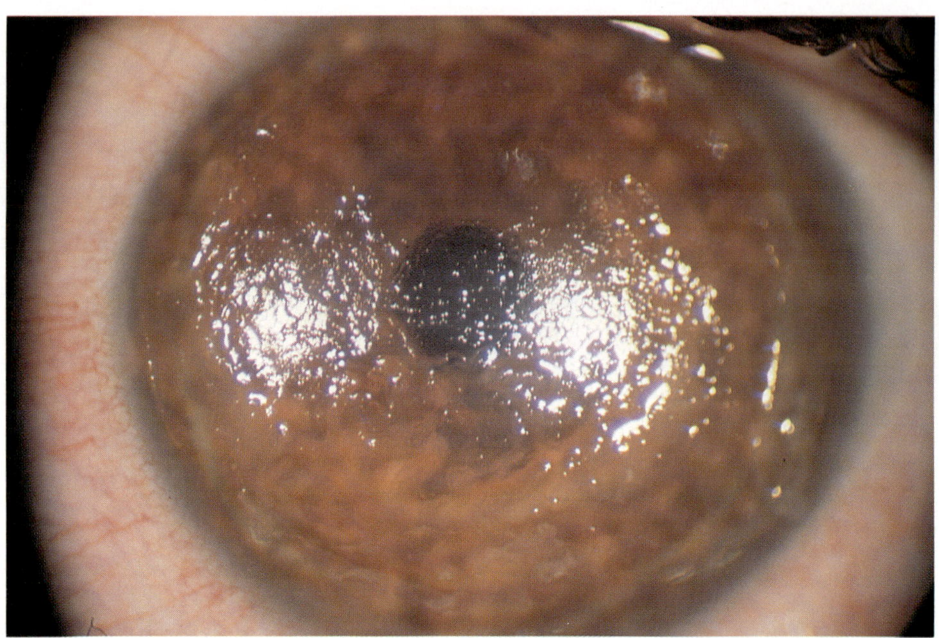

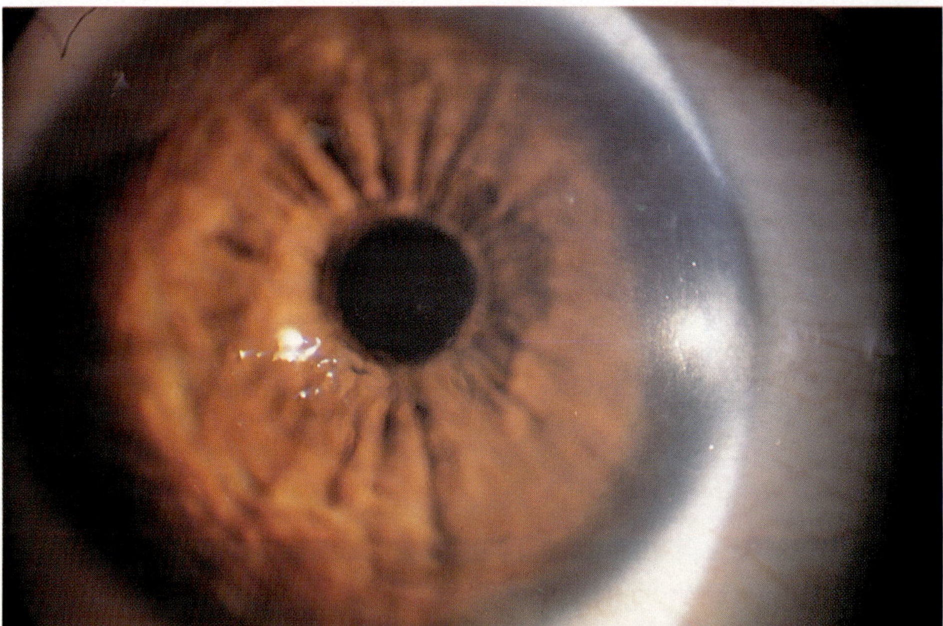

Figure 3–13 (B).   Immediately postoperatively, some dystrophic material remains and the cornea demonstrates a ground-glass appearance. **(C)** Six months postoperatively, the cornea is clear with restoration of spectacle-corrected visual acuity to 20/30 with a refraction of −2.50.

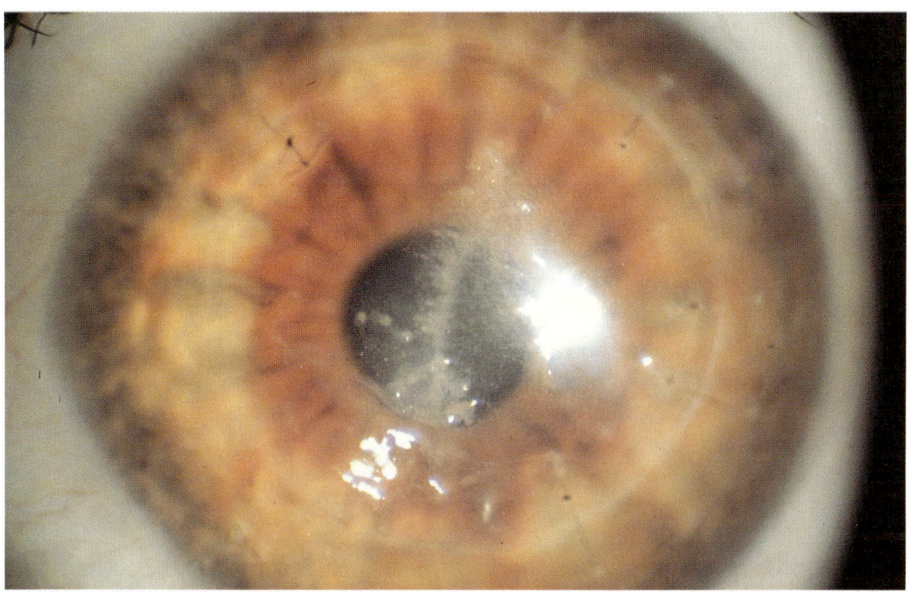

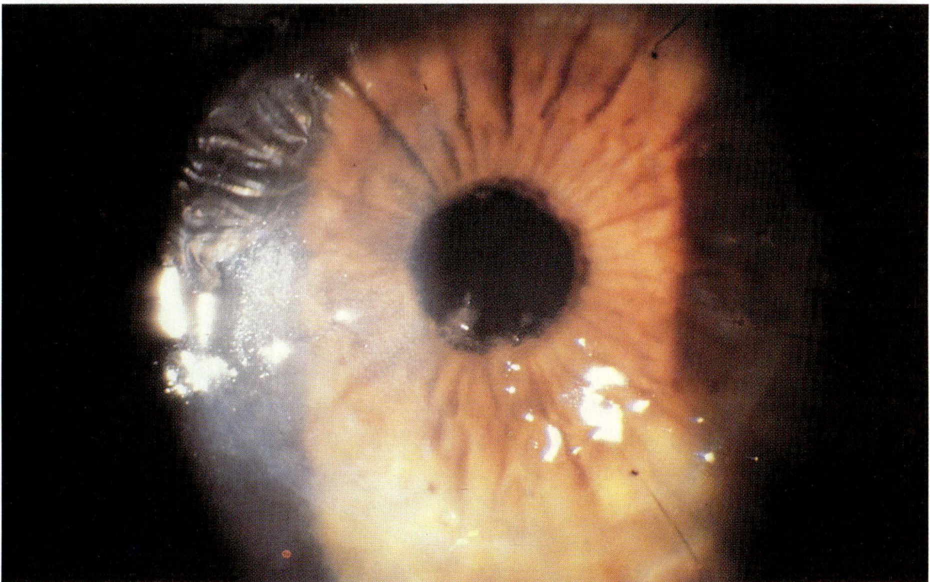

Figure 3–14.   Case 5. **(A)** A 41-year-old woman with recurrent lattice dystrophy in a corneal graft. Note the irregular corneal surface and thick ropy lattice deposits beneath the epithelium and in the superficial corneal stroma. Visual acuity is 20/80. **(B)** Following PTK, there is a small amount of residual dystrophic material with a clear and smooth central cornea. Visual acuity has improved to 20/25.

Algorithmic analysis.

Horizontal assessment and pattern. The pathology is in the central optical zone (green color code) and is segmental in its pattern.

Vertical assessment. On slit-lamp examination, the pathologic process appears to encompass the epithelium, the subepithelial area, and the superficial stroma.

Surgical therapy and outcome. The goal of the procedure in this case is three-fold: (1) clear the opacity, (2) smooth the cornea, and (3) reduce the ocular surface discomfort secondary to the irregular epithelial surface. General large area PTK using the polishing technique and masking methylcellulose was performed. The epithelium was left in place since it masked the intervening clear and smooth areas of corneal stroma. In addition, methlycellulose was placed around the elevated lattice deposits to further mask the healthy cornea as the deposits were being ablated. The patient was brought to the slit lamp many times to follow the progress of treatment in order to smooth the cornea while not removing excessive normal stromal tissue. Postoperatively, the cornea had cleared and smoothed with improvement in vision to 20/25. Patient comfort also improved.

Combined Manual Superficial Keratectomy and PTK

The rate of removal of material is dependent on its makeup. For instance, just as epithelium ablates at a rate different from stroma, similarly abnormal materials such as fibrous corneal scars and corneal dystrophic and degenerative materials may demonstrate differential ablation rates (Fig. 3–15).[13,14] Therefore, a point-and-shoot laser technique could result in an irregular surface as portions of the treated areas ablate more rapidly than others (Fig. 3–16). Calcific band keratopathy is exemplary of a corneal disorder requiring this technique (Fig. 3–17). In addition, vascularized tissue, such as a fibrovasular pannus or pterygium, is difficult to remove with the laser, since associated bleeding will block the incoming laser beam during the laser procedure. In these corneal disorders where abnormal tissue may be ablation resistant or in other situations where there is abundant deposition of abnormal material, such as in pterygia or climatic droplet keratopathy, the PTK procedure, therefore, should be combined with manual superficial keratectomy (Fig. 3–18).

In accomplishing the manual superficial keratectomy procedure as detailed above, the cleavage plane between abnormal tissue and stroma is identified by blunt dissection after initial epithelial removal; a dry cellulose sponge is a useful, atraumatic instrument for this step. The abnormal tissue is then peeled and stripped using dry sponges and fine tissue forceps. Sharp dissection may be necessary to remove firmly adherent tissue, always remaining parallel to the cleavage plane to avoid deeper stromal damage.[15,16]

After completion of manual superficial keratectomy, phototherapeutic keratectomy is accomplished using the standard techniques of the general PTK

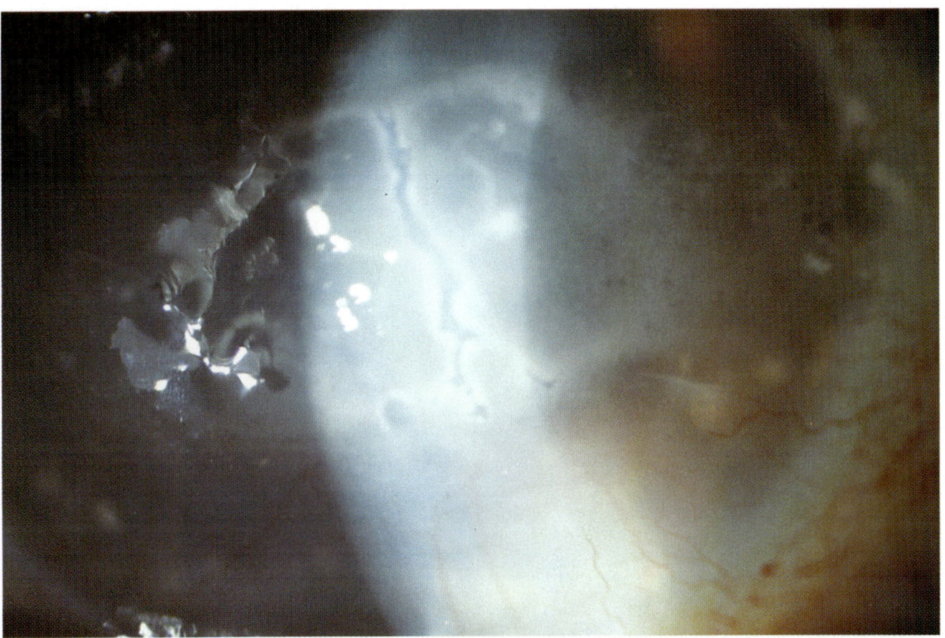

Figure 3–15.   Abundant calcium, as seen in this patient with band keratopathy, may be resistant to laser ablation and should be removed manually before PTK.

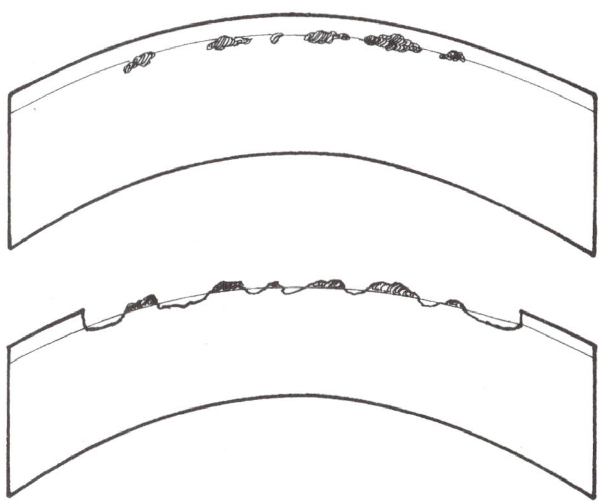

Figure 3–16.   Schematic depicting an ablation-resistant material (e.g., calcium) within the stroma leading to an irregular corneal surface after PTK.

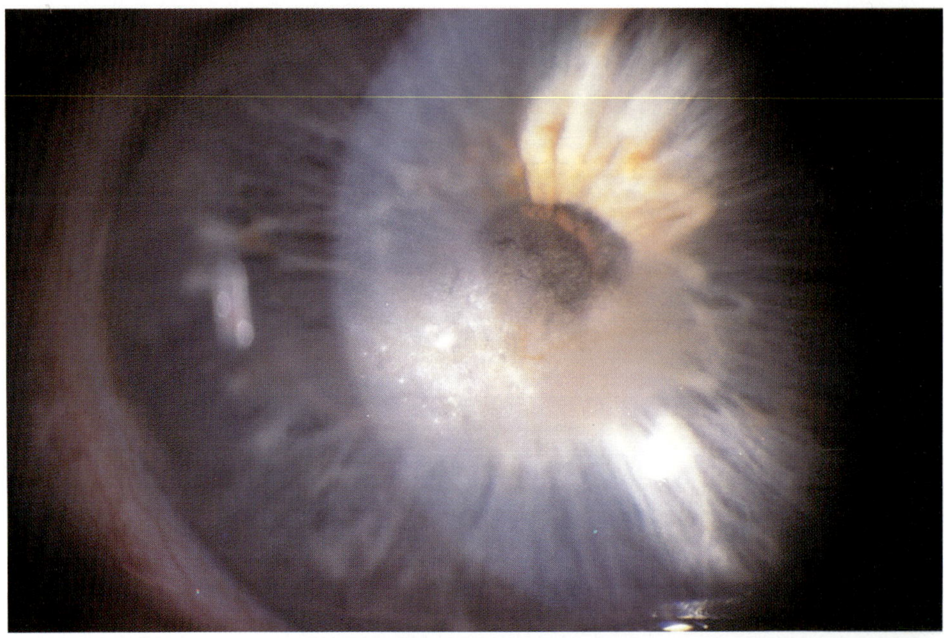

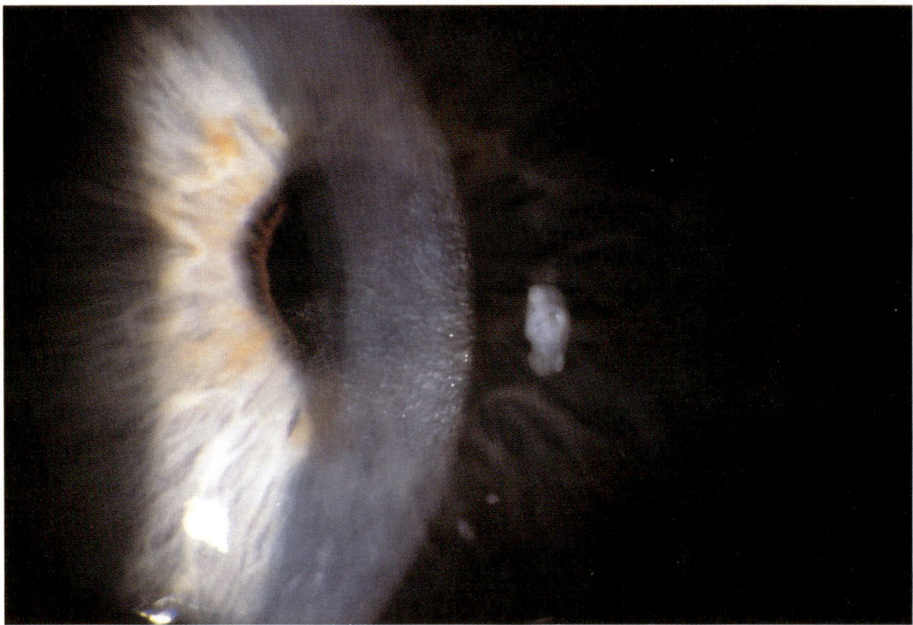

Figure 3–17. Case 6. **(A)** Preoperative appearance of a 45-year-old woman with calcific band keratopathy. Best-corrected visual acuity is counting fingers. **(B)** Three months following combined manual superficial keratectomy and PTK, the cornea is markedly clearer with improvement of visual acuity to 20/100.

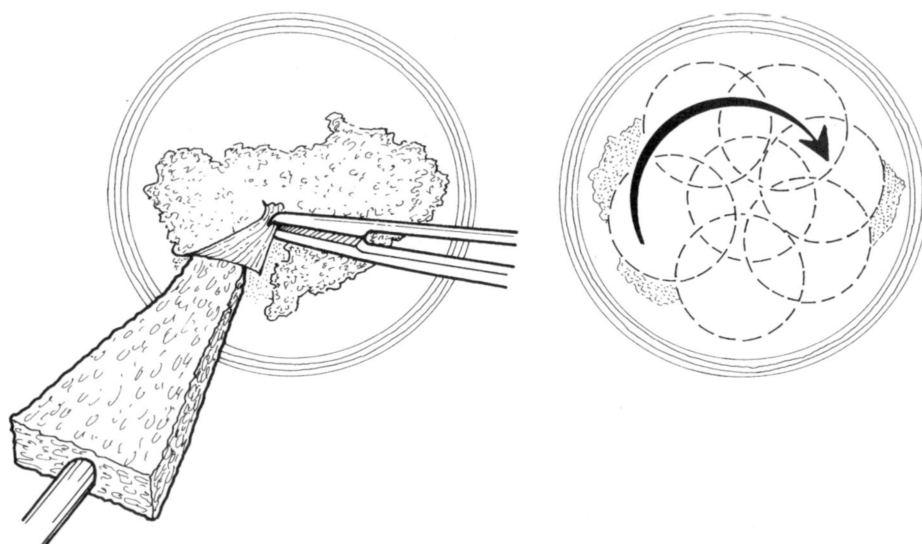

Figure 3–18.   Technique of combined manual superficial keratectomy and PTK. **(Left)** Schematic showing meticulous peeling and stripping of surface deposition, avoiding sharp dissection. **(Right)** PTK is then performed using the general large area smoothing strategy.

procedure. In cases where the corneal pathology is localized while other areas of the cornea are normal, only that area will be treated with the laser (see below). In such cases, a smaller beam diameter may be used and normal areas of the cornea may be protected by methylcellulose from unwanted ablation.

CASE 7

History and preoperative evaluation.   A 42-year-old man suffered calcific band keratopathy and cataract secondary to juvenile rheumatoid arthritis. Visual acuity was 20/200. On slit-lamp examination, abundant calcium deposition causing opacity and surface irregularity was apparent (Fig. 3–19). A cataract and posterior synechiae were also seen.

Algorithmic analysis.

HORIZONTAL ASSESSMENT AND PATTERN.   The pathology is in the central optical zone and is segmental in its pattern.

VERTICAL ASSESSMENT.   On slit-lamp examination, the pathological process appears to encompass the epithelium, the subepithelial area, and the superficial stroma.

Surgical therapy and outcome.   Manual superficial keratectomy was performed, removing much of the calcific material. At the completion of this

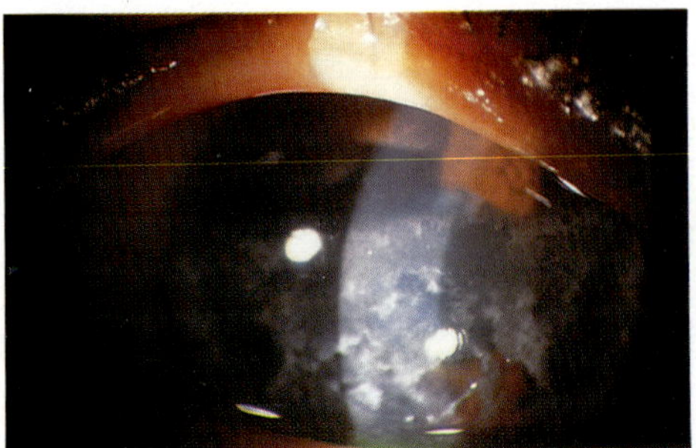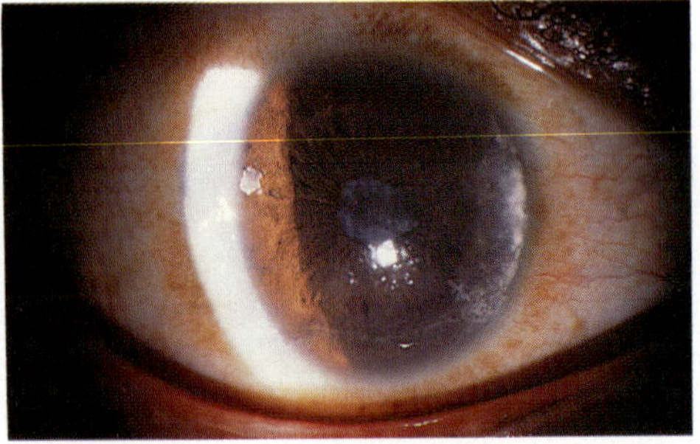

Figure 3–19.   Case 7. **(A)** Preoperative appearance of a 42-year-old man with calcific band keratopathy and cataract secondary to juvenile rheumatoid arthritis. Visual acuity is 20/200. **(B)** Following combined manual superficial keratectomy and PTK, the cornea has been cleared and smoothed with improvement in visual acuity to 20/80. After subsequent cataract extraction, visual acuity improved to 20/30.

procedure, residual calcific material remained, and the corneal surface was irregular. Standard PTK techniques using a 5 mm beam diameter and 632 laser pulses were then used to further clear and smooth the surface. Following PTK, visual acuity improved to 20/80. One month following this procedure, cataract extraction was performed and visual acuity improved to 20/30.

Focal Smoothing

Focal nodules and discrete corneal opacities may be treated directly with the excimer laser beam. For example, Salzmann's nodular degeneration may be treated, and reports have suggested the use of focal PTK for apical nodules in keratoconus patients to smooth the cornea and allow resumption of contact lens wear.[17,18] In many cases, however, such nodules can be satisfactorily removed using traditional manual superficial keratectomy techniques (see Chapter 2), or manual keratectomy can be used as an adjunct to focal PTK (Fig. 3–20).

In performing focal PTK, the amount of elevation is first estimated by slit-lamp examination. In some cases, an optical pachymeter may be used to directly measure the elevation. The approximate number of anticipated laser pulses can then be calculated (No. of pulses = elevation in microns × 4). The epithelium over the area to be treated is manually removed, again with blunt dissection. The surrounding epithelium, however, is left intact to shield normal corneal stroma from ablation. Surrounding normal areas may also be masked with methycellulose. The laser spot size is chosen to coincide with the nodule being treated. The laser is aimed at the nodule and treatment then applied to smooth the elevated area. The patient is examined frequently at the slit lamp until the surface is smooth. Care is taken to avoid overtreatment with consequent crater formation on the corneal surface.

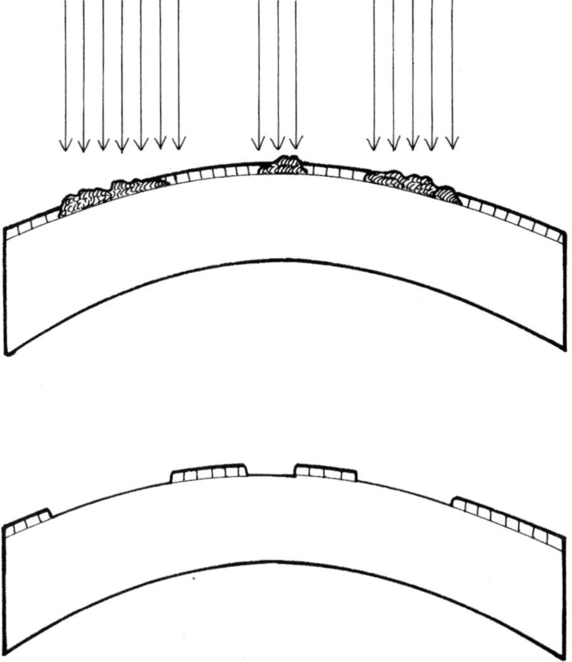

Figure 3–20.   Technique of focal smoothing using the excimer laser. The laser beam diameter is adjusted per the size of the nodular elevation. Epithelium is left in place over normal areas of cornea, protecting such areas from ablation.

CASE 8

History and preoperative evaluation.   A 55-year-old man presented with an elevated plaque-like fibrous scar secondary to trauma (Fig. 3–21). Uncorrected visual acuity was 20/100 and spectacle-corrected visual acuity was 20/32. The patient complained of severe glare symptoms.

Algorithmic analysis.

HORIZONTAL ASSESSMENT AND PATTERN.   The pathology is peripheral, and it is segmental in its pattern.

VERTICAL ASSESSMENT.   The scar is elevated. It appears to go to the level of Bowman's layer.

Surgical therapy and outcome.   Epithelium was removed with dry cellulose sponges over the area of the fibrous scar. Blunt dissection with 0.12 mm forceps and dry cellulose sponges was rewarded by stripping of the nodule. A 5 mm PTK beam was then used to polish the remaining surface until the contour was appropriate. One year following treatment, the visual axis was cleared with improvement of uncorrected visual acuity to 20/50 and best-

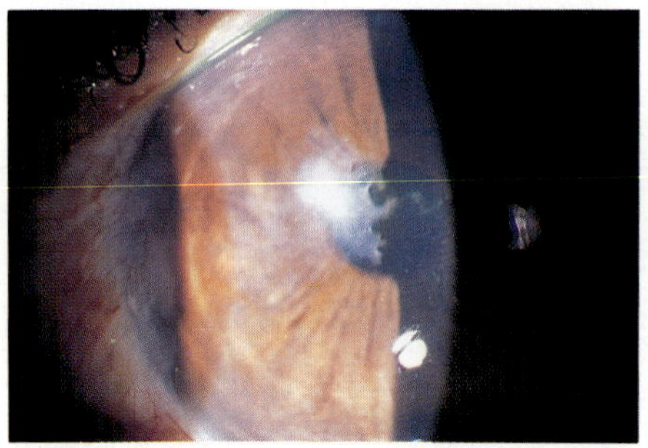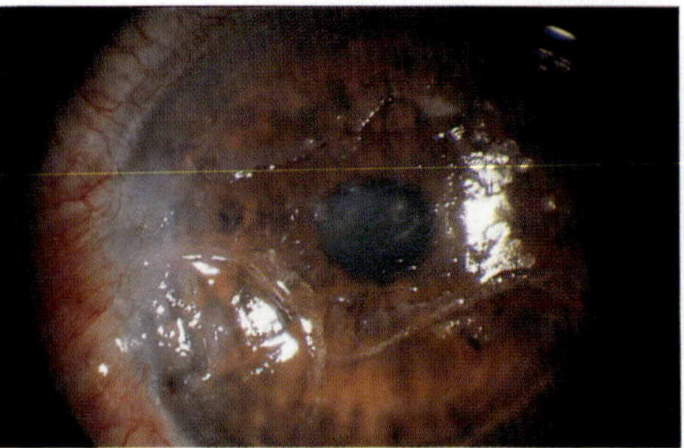

Figure 3–21.   Case 8. **(A)** Preoperative appearance of a 55-year-old man with an elevated, plaquelike, fibrous scar secondary to trauma. Uncorrected visual acuity was 20/100, and spectacle-corrected visual acuity was 20/32. The patient complained of severe glare symptoms. **(B)** Immediately following focal PTK treatment, the visual axis is cleared with ultimate improvement of uncorrected visual acuity to 20/50 and spectacle-corrected visual acuity to 20/20 with marked decrease in glare symptoms.

corrected spectacle visual acuity to 20/20. The patient noted a marked decrease in his glare symptoms.

CASE 9

History and preoperative evaluation.   An 80-year-old man with Salzmann's nodular degeneration complained of monocular diplopia and photophobia (Fig. 3–22). On examination, the monocular diplopia disappeared when the nodules were covered by the edge of a card. Visual acuity was 20/40. On slit-lamp examination, two nodules were present, measuring approximately 2.0 and 1.5 mm, respectively. Videokeratoscopy demonstrated focal irregularity superiorly at rings 1–4 overlying a corneal nodule and steepening over the nodules.

Algorithmic analysis.

Horizontal assessment and pattern.   The pathology is in the paracentral zone, and it is nodular in its pattern.

Vertical assessment.   The nodules were elevated and appeared to go down to the level of Bowman's layer.

Surgical therapy and outcome.   The epithelium was removed with dry cellulose sponges over the nodules themselves, but left in place over the areas of clear cornea. For the first nodule, the laser beam diameter was set for 2.0 mm and the laser was delivered for 253 pulses until the level of the nodule was lowered to the normal corneal surface. A 2.0 mm beam and 217 pulses were used for the second nodule. Following focal PTK, the monocular diplopia and photophobia resolved. The videokeratoscope image was more regular, and the corresponding topographic map showed marked improvement in the

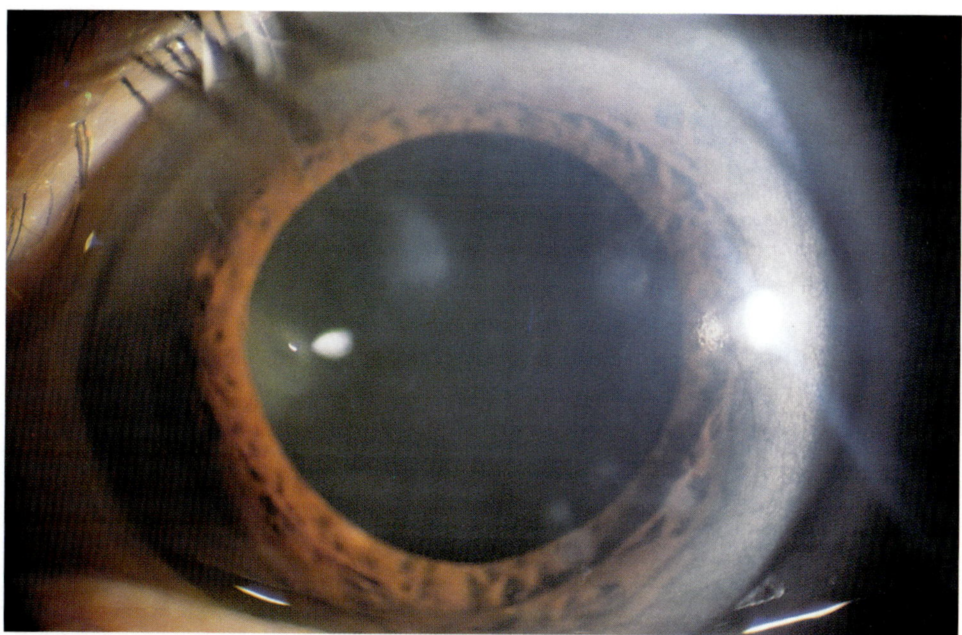

Figure 3–22.   Case 9. **(A)** An 80-year-old man with Salzmann's nodular degeneration complained of monocular diplopia and photophobia. Visual acuity is 20/40. **(B)** Following focal excimer laser smoothing of the superior nodules, the monocular diplopia and photophobia have resolved. Visual acuity is 20/25. **(C, top left)** Videokeratoscope image before PTK shows focal irregularity superiorly at rings 1–4 overlying corneal nodule. **(C, top right)** Corresponding topographic map demonstrating corneal steepening over the nodule. **(C, bottom left)** Following focal PTK, the videokeratoscope image is more regular. **(C, bottom right)** Corresponding topographic map shows marked improvement in the corneal steepening with decrease in irregular astigmatism. *(Continued on following page)*

corneal steepening with a decrease in irregular astigmatism. Postoperative visual acuity was 20/25.

CASE 10

History and preoperative evaluation.   A 64-year-old man was seen with a complaint of poor vision and ocular surface discomfort of the left eye (Fig. 3–23). On examination, spectacle-corrected visual acuity was 20/50, improving to 20/40 with a rigid contact lens. A 5.0 mm elevated nodule was seen in the superonasal quadrant of the cornea.

Algorithmic analysis.

Horizontal assessment and pattern.   A nodular pattern is seen in the periphery of the cornea.

Vertical assessment.   The pathology is at the level of Bowman's layer and the anterior stroma.

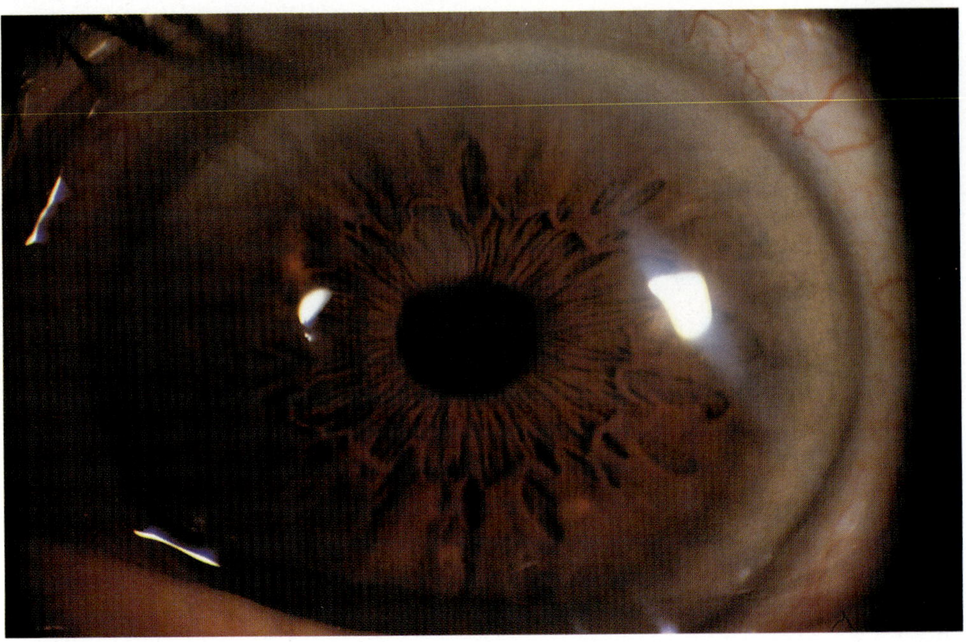

Figure 3–22 (B)

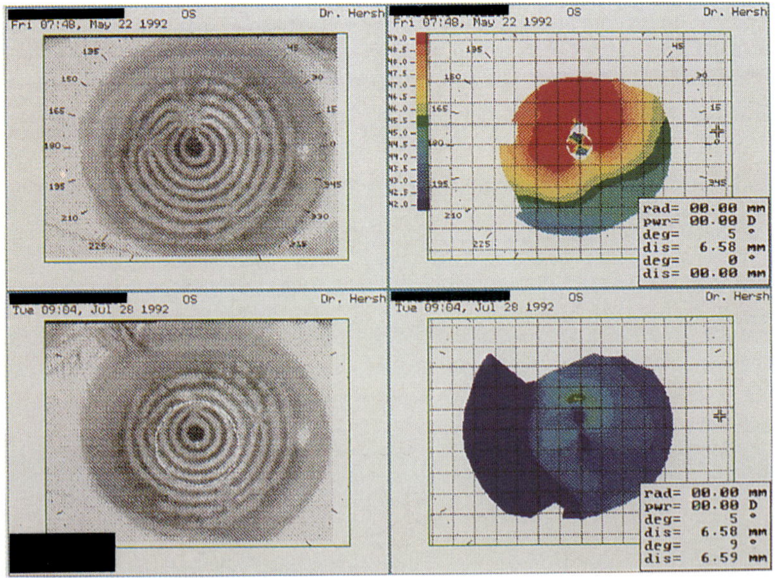

Figure 3–22 (C)

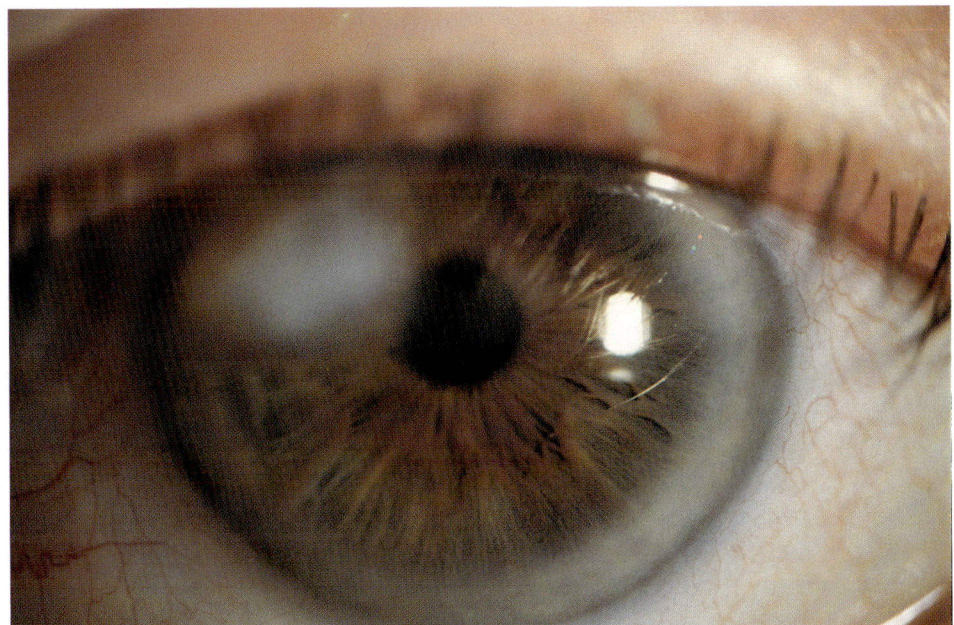

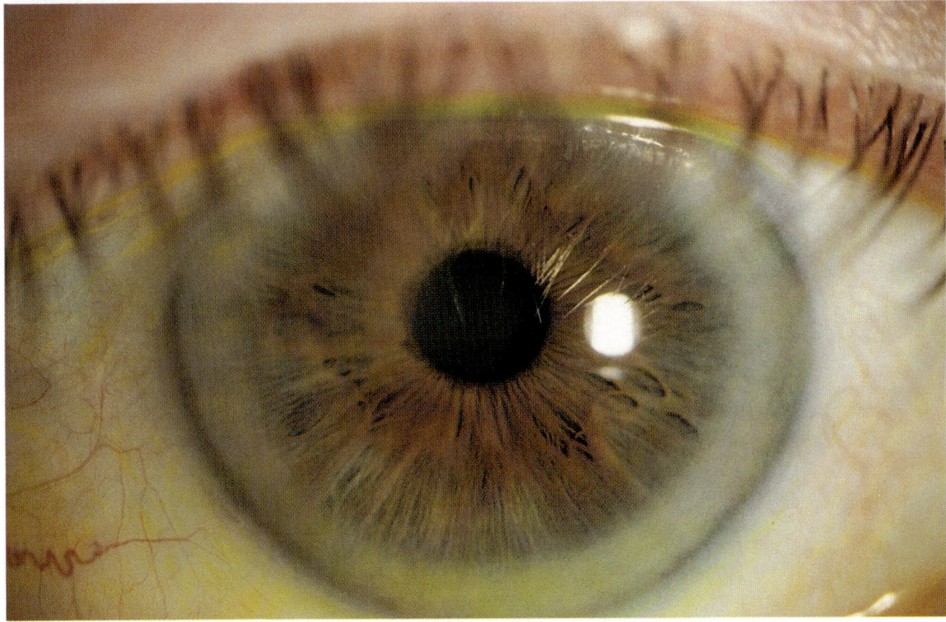

Figure 3–23. Case 10. **(A)** A 64-year-old man was seen with a complaint of poor vision and ocular surface discomfort of the left eye. On examination, spectacle-corrected visual acuity is 20/50, improving to 20/40 with a rigid contact lens. A 5.0 mm elevated nodule is seen in the superonasal quadrant of the cornea. **(B)** Following focal PTK, the cornea has cleared, spectacle-corrected visual acuity has improved to 20/25, and the eye is comfortable.

Surgical therapy and outcome.   Manual stripping of the nodule was attempted without success since a cleavage plane over Bowman's layer was difficult to obtain. Therefore, focal PTK was performed. The epithelium was removed with dry cellulose sponges over the nodule and left in place over the areas of clear cornea. The laser beam diameter was set for 4.0 mm, and approximately 100 laser pulses were applied. Further manual stripping was then rewarded by removal of much of the remaining nodule from the corneal surface. Additional laser was performed after methylcellulose 1% had been applied to further smooth the corneal surface in the area of the nodule. Following focal PTK, there remained only a faint haze in the area of the previous nodule. Monocular diplopia and photophobia had resolved.

Superficial Scar Removal

Focal superficial corneal scars may be ablated with careful attention to the minimization of postoperative corneal topographic and refractive changes (usually hyperopic shifts; see Chapter 6), which may result from stromal tissue removal. The treatment of corneal scars thus exemplifies the importance of clearly defining therapeutic goals, identifying coincidental clinical effects, and adhering to meticulous technique. Although scars within the corneal stroma usually can be easily ablated with the excimer laser, perturbations in the postoperative corneal surface topography may require a rigid contact lens to achieved best possible vision. In some cases, residual topographic irregularity may actually decrease uncorrected vision while vision with a rigid contact lens may improve. Similarly, refractive shifts may result in postoperative anisometropia and lead to a clinically unsatisfactory result.

In general, only superficial scars (<100 µm) should be treated. Optical or ultrasonic pachymetry may be helpful to judge the depth of the scar and overall corneal thickness.[19] Corneas that are thin should not be treated, since additional tisssue removal may make the cornea ectatic or may further distort the corneal surface.

TECHNIQUE 1

If the corneal epithelial surface is smooth, the epithelium overlying the scar is left in place and removed with the laser. As noted earlier, epithelium may naturally fill in surface irregularities of the scarred stroma, thus leading to a smoother surface after PTK. Any irregularities that subsequently develop during treatment are smoothed with methylcellulose 1%. In the first technique, removal of the scar is combined with active blending of the ablation zone borders by rotating the patient's head gently during treatment as in the general PTK technique (Fig. 3–24). A large area beam (>5.0 mm) is generally used to avoid focal distortions of the corneal stroma as a consequence of uneven ablation with a small beam. In addition, actual tissue ablation should be minimized to avoid postoperative corneal surface distortion; it is unnecessary to remove the entire scar from the cornea. Rather, "debulking" of the scar may give a visually satisfactory result. The amount of tissue ablation

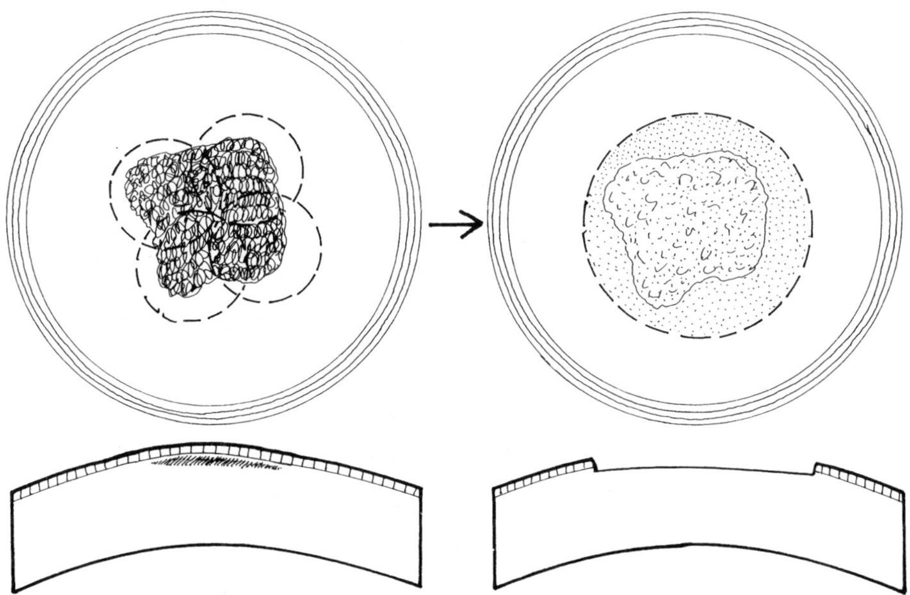

Figure 3–24.   Technique of superficial scar removal using the polishing technique. Schematic showing annular motion of eye under the laser beam creating a blend zone around the area of the scar. Treatment should be minimized to avoid postoperative changes in the corneal topography.

can be monitored by the sound and appearance of the ablation as previously described. Moreover, the patient may be brought frequently to the slit lamp to evaluate the necessity of additional laser treatment.

CASES 11 AND 12

History and preoperative evaluation.   A 50-year-old woman (Case 11) had a superficial scar secondary to previous herpetic keratitis (Fig. 3–25). Uncorrected visual acuity is count fingers, and best spectacle and contact lens visual acuity is 20/100.

Algorithmic analysis.

Horizontal assessment and pattern.   The pathology is centrally located.

Vertical assessment.   The scar involves Bowman's layer and the anterior corneal stroma.

Surgical therapy and outcome.   The epithelium was left in place since it appeared relatively smooth. Epithelial removal was noted by the change in the blue fluorescence pattern. A polishing technique was used. Three months

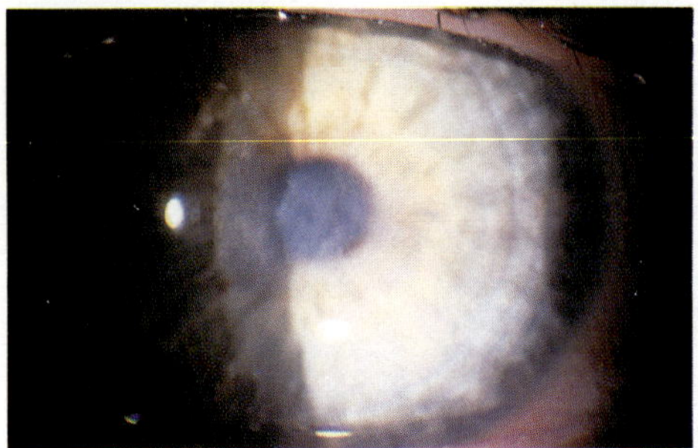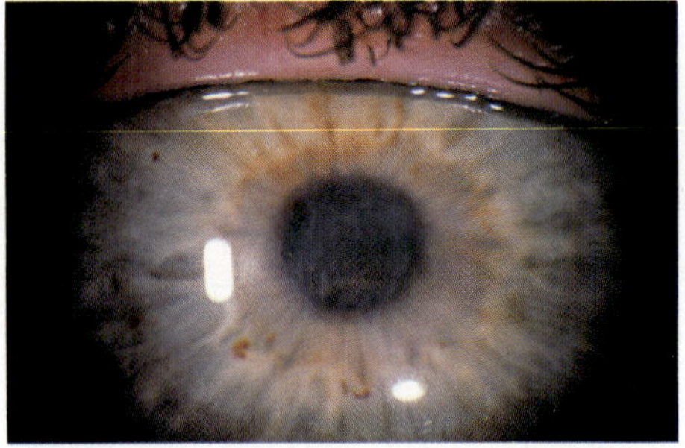

Figure 3–25.   Case 11. **(A)** Preoperative appearance of a 50-year-old woman who underwent PTK for the removal of a superficial scar secondary to previous herpes keratitis. Uncorrected visual acuity is counting fingers, and best-corrected spectacle and contact lens vision is 20/100. **(B)** Three months following PTK, uncorrected visual acuity has improved to 20/200 and spectacle-corrected visual acuity has remained 20/100 secondary to residual astigmatism. Visual acuity with a rigid contact lens has improved to 20/40.

following PTK, uncorrected visual acuity improved to 20/200 and spectacle-corrected visual acuity remained 20/100 secondary to residual astigmatism (see Chapter 6). Visual acuity with a rigid contact lens improved to 20/40. However, the patient was unable to tolerate long-term contact lens wear and subsequently underwent penetrating keratoplasty.

TECHNIQUE 2

In this technique of scar removal, a wide beam diameter (usually ≥6.0 mm) is used to directly ablate the scar without movement of the patient's head. The treatment is centered on the pupil rather than the scar itself to avoid postoperative optical zone edge effects.[5] The number of pulses may be estimated by the depth of the corneal scar (No. of pulses = depth of scar in microns × 4), but should be minimized to avoid refractive shifts. Again, the entire thickness of the scar need not be removed for visual improvement. Epithelial removal is monitored by its blue fluorescence and usually requires 150–200 pulses.

Upon satisfactory removal of the scar, the center of the treatment zone is then masked with a drop of methylcellulose 2.5%. This should be applied to mask the central 5.0 mm, leaving a peripheral annulus exposed to the laser beam. A sterile filter paper or soft contact lens punched to 5.0 mm can also be used to mask the central cornea. Additional treatment (approximately 50–100 pulses) is then applied to create a peripheral annulus with the goal of preventing hyperopic refractive shifts (Figs. 3–26, 3–27; case 12; see Chapter 6). When future excimer lasers are able to perform hyperopic corrections, it is possible that a hyperopic correction may be used as part of the PTK procedure to avoid corneal flattening.

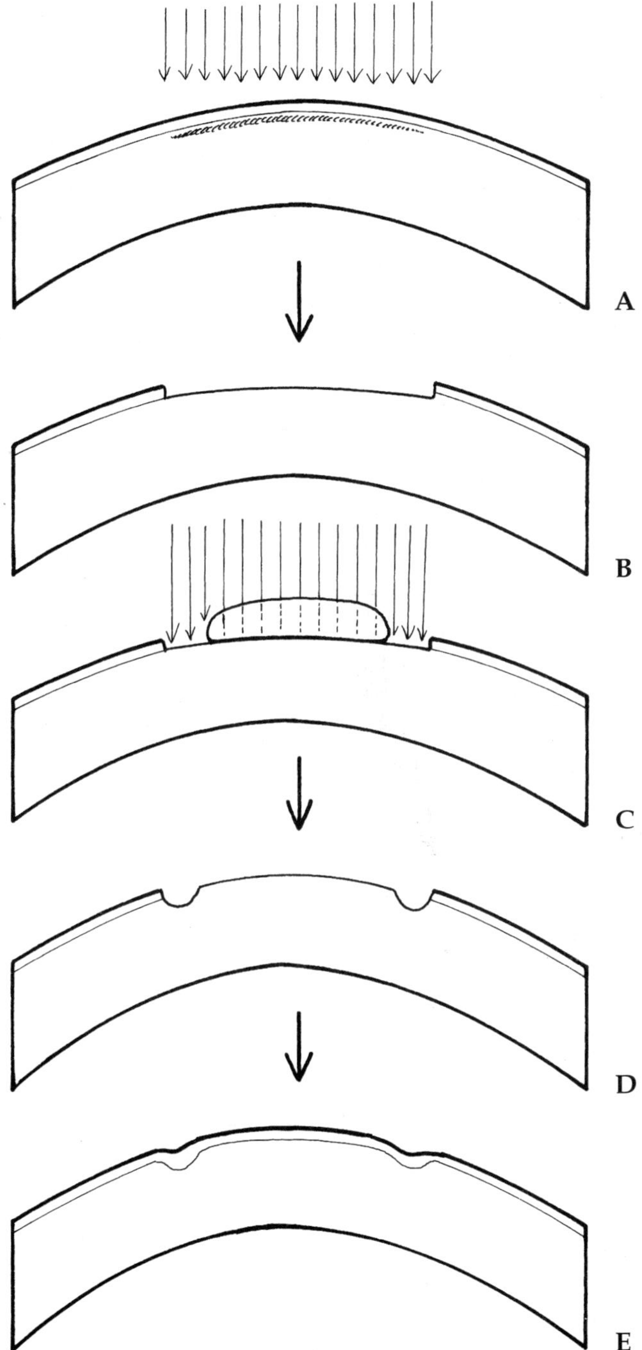

Figure 3–26. Technique of superficial scar removal using direct laser application with peripheral annulus. **(A,B)** Direct application of laser to scar using wide beam diameter (usually ≥6.0 mm). Laser beam is centered over the pupil. **(C,D)** Methylcellulose 2.5% (or a prepared filter paper or contact lens mask) is used to protect center of cornea while periphery of the beam ablates an approximately 1 mm surrounding annulus to form a blend zone into untreated cornea. **(E)** After epithelium heals, corneal flattening is mitigated by relative steepening of the corneal conture.

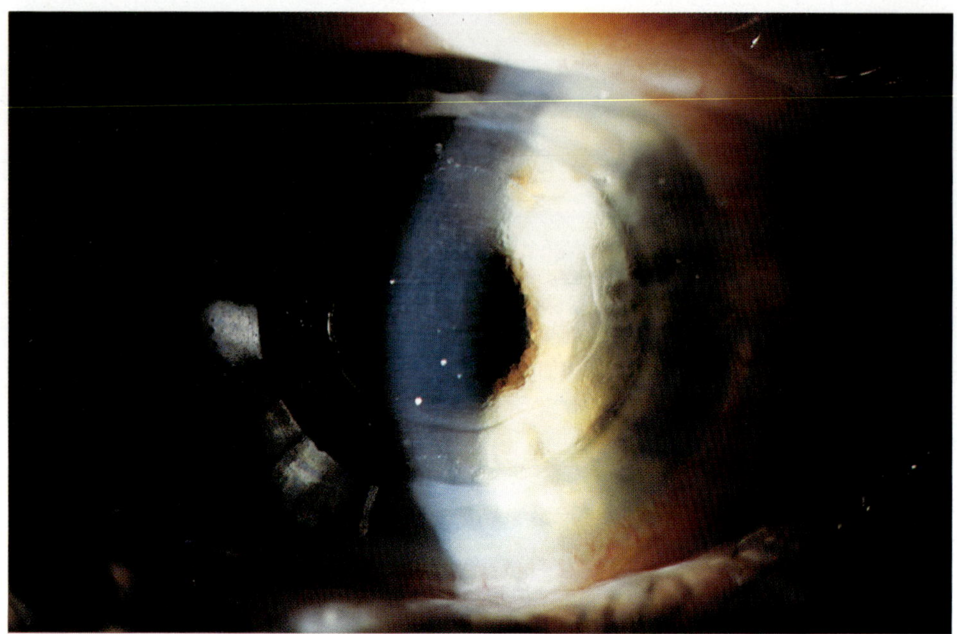

Figure 3–27.   Case 12. Immediately following treatment of a central corneal scar in a 64-year-old man showing clear cornea with an annulus of additional treatment to prevent hyperopic shift.

Epithelial Basement Membrane Dystrophy and Recurrent Epithelial Erosion Syndrome

Success in the treatment of recurrent erosion syndrome is likely due to meticulous smoothing and cleaning of the subepithelial corneal surface affording a substrate conducive to epithelial migration and adhesion.[20] This has been shown to be effective in the case of recurrent epithelial erosions caused by epithelial basement membrane dystrophy and may be useful for other causes of epithelial dysadherence.[21] The putative mechanism of PTK in such circumstances is in contrast to the anterior stromal puncture procedure where focal cicatrization is thought to mediate improved epithelial adherence (Fig. 3–28).

Dysadherent epithelium overlying the area of a recalcitrant recurrent erosion is carefully removed using a dry cellulose sponge as the primary instrument and the back of a scarifier blade only if necessary. Underlying reduplicated basement membrane or cellular debris is then carefully stripped to leave a smooth surface. Forceps (0.12 mm) may be useful in this stripping technique.[22] Spot size is determined by the area of abnormality to be treated. Approximately 15 pulses are directly applied, resulting in a nominal ablation of 3.75 μm (Fig. 3–29). In cases of larger areas to be treated, approximately 15 pulses per unit area are applied, the patient's head being rotated to uni-

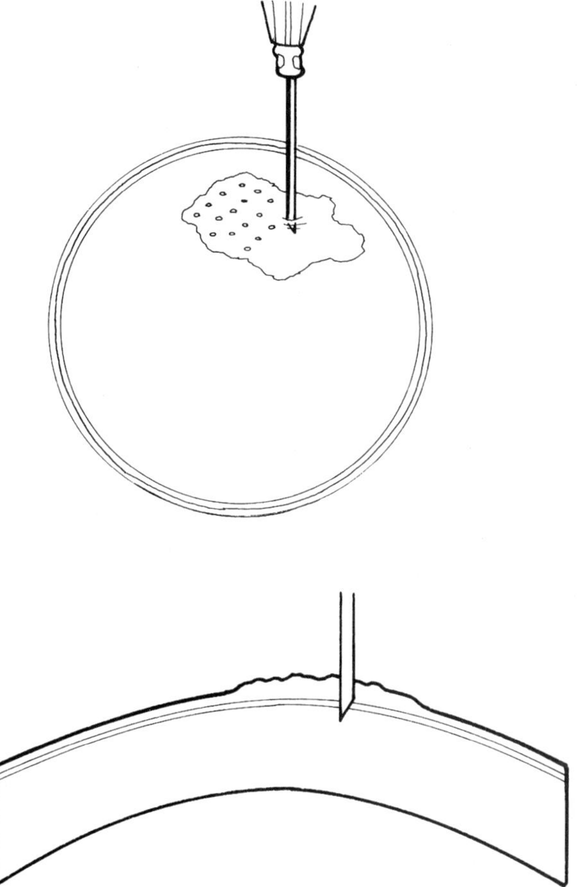

Figure 3–28. Anterior stromal puncture. Multiple superficial punctures with a disposable (No. 20) needle are used to stimulate microcicatrization between epithelium, Bowman's layer, and anterior stroma.

formly distribute the ablation. This technique is thought to meticulously clean and smooth the corneal surface, leaving both an optically clear cornea and a smooth stromal substrate for subsequent re-epithelialization. Moreover, the minimal number of laser pulses necessary likely leads to little change in corneal topography or refractive error.[21]

CASE 13

History and preoperative evaluation. A 26-year-old woman with myopia of − 24.0 diopters presented with a recurrent corneal epithelial erosion following many years of rigid contact lens wear (Fig. 3–30). This was recalcitrant to treatment with lubrication and a bandage soft contact lens. It prevented

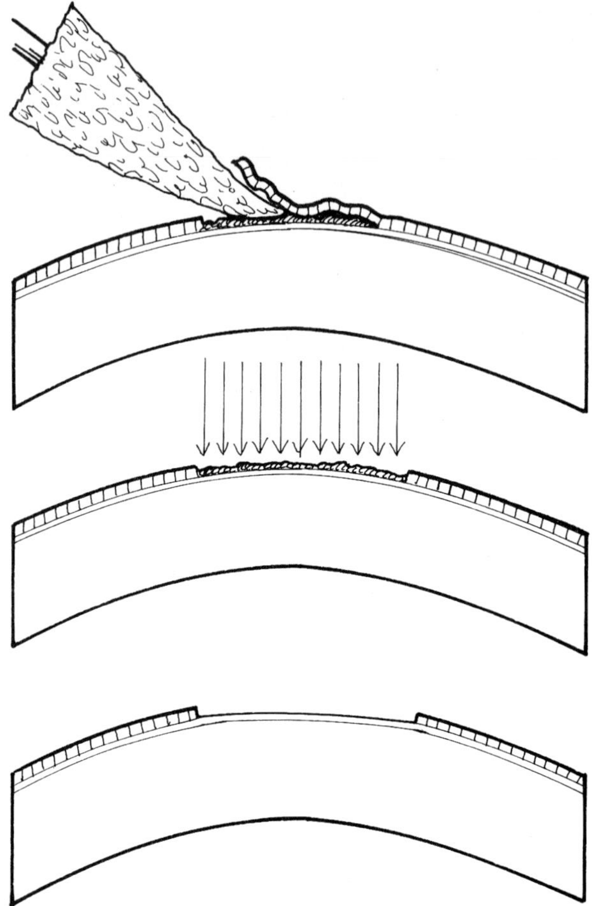

Figure 3–29.   Technique of PTK for recurrent corneal epithelial erosions second-ary to epithelial basement membrane abnormalities. **(Top)** Dysadherent epithelium is gently stripped with a dry cellulose sponge. **(Middle)** The excimer laser beam is applied focally for approximately 15 pulses for each unit area. **(Bottom)** At the conclusion of the procedure, Bowman's layer is smooth without abnormal over-lying basement membrane, affording an appropriate substrate for subsequent re-epithelialization.

her from successfully wearing her contact lenses, which she required for good vision.

Surgical therapy and outcome.   Under local anaesthesia, the area of disadherent epithelium was debrided with dry cellulose sponges. The area measured approximately 3 mm. The surface was dried, and a 15 pulse PTK treatment with a beam diameter of 3.5 was undertaken. Spectacle-corrected visual acu-ity improved to 20/25, and the patient resumed contact lens wear.

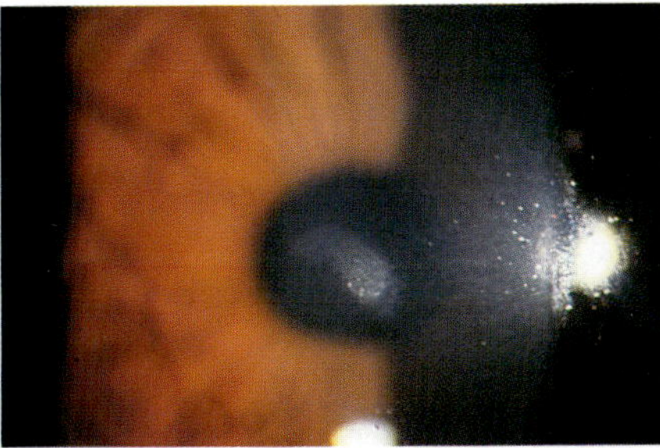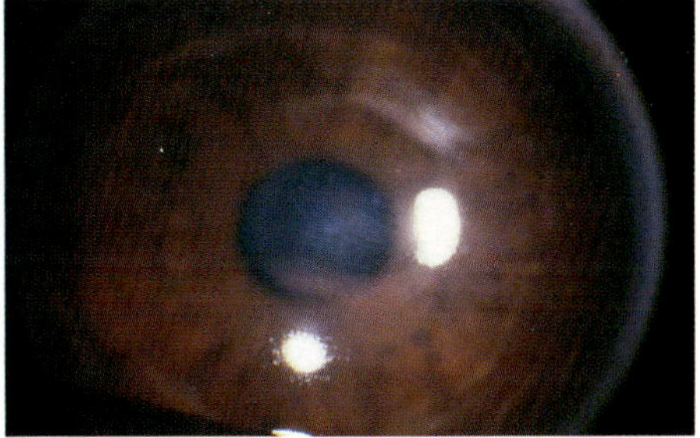

Figure 3–30.   Case 13. **(A)** Preoperative appearance of a 26-year-old woman with recurrent erosion syndrome. Note abnormal basement membrane and superficial scarring overlying the visual axis. The area partially stains with fluorescein. **(B)** Following a 15 pulse PTK treatment, the epithelium is firmly adherent, smooth, and lustrous. Best-corrected visual acuity improved from 20/125 to 20/25, and the patient was able to resume contact lens wear.

Postoperative Management

Postoperative care is directed toward facilitating re-epithelialization, minimizing inflammation and scarring, and avoiding infection (see Chapter 5). In general, the eye is patched or a therapeutic soft contact lens is applied. A topical antibiotic and corticosteroid are generally used. Oral analgesic agents are given as necessary, and topical nonsteroidal anti-inflammatory agents may be used judiciously for pain control. Following superficial keratectomy and PTK, patients usually do not have severe discomfort.

Nonpreserved lubricants are used as needed. A therapeutic contact lens may be continued if epithelialization is delayed. Topical antibiotics are continued until epithelialization is complete and continued in the presence of a therapeutic soft contact lens. A corticosteroid drop is generally used four times daily and tapered by one drop each month to decrease the risk of inflammation and scarring. A mild steroid such as fluorometholone 0.1% may be used in most cases. In the presence or likelihood of more profound surface inflammation, a stronger corticosteroid such as prednisolone acetate 1% may be used. Following treatment for epithelial basement membrane dystrophy, corticosteroids are generally not used since treatment is minimal. In patients treated for scarring secondary to herpes simplex keratitis, oral acyclovir (400 mg three times daily) and topical antiviral agents may be administered perioperatively to avoid reactivation of the virus.[23]

Conclusions

A number of surgical strategies are available with the PTK procedure. The surgeon must practice careful case selection, choose an appropriate surgical strategy tailored to the individual patient problem, and properly execute the procedure to optimize clinical outcomes.

References

1. Kenyon KR, Tseng SCG. Limbal autograft transplantation for ocular surface disorders. Ophthalmology 1989;96:709–723.
2. Kornmehl EW, Steinert RF, Puliafito CA. A comparative study of masking fluids for excimer laser phototherapeutic keratectomy. Arch Ophthalmol. 1991;109:860–863.
3. Englanoff JS, Kolahdouz-Isfahani AH, Moreira H, Cheung DT, Nimni ME, Trokel SL, McDonnell PJ. In situ collagen gel mold as an aid in excimer laser superficial keratectomy. Ophthalmology 1992;99:1201–1208.
4. Fasano AP, Moreira H, McDonnell PJ, Sinbawy A. Excimer laser smoothing of a reproducible model of anterior corneal surface irregularity. Ophthalmology 1991;98:1783–1785.
5. Schwartz-Goldstein B, Hersh PS. Summit PRK Topography Study Group. Corneal topography of phase III excimer laser photorefractive keratectomy: optical zone centration analysis. Ophthalmology 1995;102:951–962.
6. Hersh PS, Spinak A, Garrana R, Mayers M. Excimer laser phototherapeutic keratectomy: strategies and results. Refract Corneal Surg 1993;9:S90–S95.
7. Tuft S, Al-Dhahir R, Dyer P, Zehao Z. Characterization of the fluorescence spectra produced by excimer laser irradiation of the cornea. Invest Ophthalmol Vis Sci 1990;31:1512–1518.
8. Gibralter R, Trokel SL. Correction of irregular astigmatism with the excimer laser. Ophthalmology 1994;101:1310–1315.
9. Munnerlyn CR, Koons SJ, Marshall J. Photorefractive keratectomy: a technique for laser refractive surgery. J Cat Refract Surg. 1988;14:46–52.
10. Sher N, Bowers RA, Zabel RW, Frantz JM, Eifferman RA, Brown DC, Rowsey JJ, Parker P, Chen V, Lindstrom RL. Clinical use of the 193-nm excimer laser in the treatment of corneal scars. Arch Ophthalmol 1991;109:491–498.
11. Stark WJ, Chanon W et al. Clinical follow-up of 193 nm ArF excimer laser photokeratectomy. Ophthalmology 1992;99:805–812.
12. Sher NA, Bowers RA, Zabel RW et al. Clinical use of the 193-nm excimer laser in the treatment of corneal scars. Arch Ophthalmol 1991;109:491–498.
13. McDonnell JM, Garbus JJ, McDonnell PJ. Unsuccessful excimer laser phototherapeutic keratectomy. Arch Ophthalmol 1992;110:977–979.
14. Binder PS, Anderson JA, Rock ME, Vrabec M. Human excimer laser keratectomy. Clinical and histopathologic correlations. Ophthalmology 1994;101:979–989.
15. Hersh PS. Ophthalmic Surgical Procedures. Boston: Little, Brown & Co. 1988:221–225.
16. Hersh PS, Kenyon KR. Anterior segment reconstruction following ocular trauma. In Shingleton BJ, Hersh PS, Kenyon KR (eds): Eye Trauma. St. Louis: Mosby–YearBook, 1991:176.
17. Steinert RF, Puliafito CA. Excimer laser phototherapeutic keratectomy for a corneal nodule. Refract Corneal Surg 1990;6:352.
18. Ward MA, Artunduaga G, Thompson KP, Wilson LA, Stulting RD. Phototherapeutic keratectomy for the treatment of nodular subepithelial corneal scars in patients with keratoconus who are contact lens intolerant. CLAO J 1995;21:130–132.
19. Reinstein DZ, Aslanides IM, Silverman RH, Asbell PA, Coleman DJ. High frequency ultrasound corneal pachymetry in the assessment of corneal scars for therapeutic planning. CLAO J 1994;20:198–203.
20. Dausch D, Landesz M, Klein R, Schroder E. Phototherapeutic keratectomy in recurrent corneal epithelial erosion. J Refract Corneal Surg 1993;9:419–424.
21. John ME, Van Der Karr MA, Noblitt RL, Boleyn KL. Excimer laser phototherapeutic keratectomy for treatment of recurrent corneal erosion. J Cataract Refract Surg 1994;20:179–182.
22. Kenyon KR, Wagoner MD. Conjunctival and corneal injuries. In Shingleton BJ, Hersh PS, Kenyon KR (eds): Eye Trauma. St. Louis: Mosby–YearBook, 1991:70–71.
23. Vrabec MP, Durrie DS, Chase DS. Recurrence of herpes simplex after excimer laser keratectomy. Am J Ophthalmol 1992;114:96–97.
24. Wagoner MD, Waller SG. Treatment of paracentral corneal scar-induced astigmatism with manual superficial keratectomy. Saudi J Ophthamology 1996;10:31–35.
25. Hersh, PS, Shah S. Corneal topography of 6 mm photorefractive keratectomy. Ophthamology 1997;104:1330–1342.

4

Clinical Results

The definition of success in an excimer laser PTK may vary considerably depending on the corneal disorder and goal of the treatment. Therefore, this chapter reviews results from selected clinical trials to give an overview of results that can be anticipated. Some of the most important "results" of PTK are the side effects and complications arising from the procedure. These are discussed in Chapters 5 and 6.

Study 1

Study Design

In a single center study[1] performed in a university-based cornea practice, with surgery perfomed by one of the authors (PH), a consecutive series of 28 eyes of 26 patients underwent the PTK for one of five general categories of corneal disorders: (1) diffuse superficial opacities and irregularities (e.g., corneal dystrophies); (2) diffuse depositions and excrescences (e.g., band keratopathy); (3) focal excresences and nodules such a Salzmann's nodular degeneration; (4) superficial corneal stromal scars; and (5) epithelial basement membrane dystrophy with recurrent epithelial erosions or visual disability. Patient age ranged from 26 to 81 years; the mean age was 51 years. Follow up ranged from 6 to 30 months; the average was 1 year. Preoperative diagnoses are listed in Table 4–1. Indications for treatment included poor best-corrected spectacle visual acuity, glare and photophobia, ocular surface discomfort, recurrent epithelial erosions, and monocular diplopia.

Phototherapeutic keratectomy was performed with the Summit OmniMed/ExciMed excimer laser system (Summit Technology, Inc., Wal-

Table 4–1.   Study 1: Preoperative Diagnoses

Preoperative Diagnosis	No. of eyes
Corneal scarring	8
Salzmann's degeneration	4
Reis-Buckler's dystrophy	5
Lattice dystrophy	1
Band keratopathy	3
Recurrent erosion syndrome	5
Contact lens induced keratopathy	1
Epithelial basement membrane dystrophy	1

Source: Reprinted with permission from Hersh et al.[1] Courtesy of *Ophthalmology.*

tham, MA). Laser parameters included a repetition rate of 10 Hz, fluence of 180 mj/cm^2, and pulse duration of 14 ns, resulting in an estimated ablation rate of corneal stromal tissue of 0.25 μm per pulse. Beam size was variable from 1.5 to 6.0 mm.

Visual acuity was measured on a logMAR scale.[2] Computer-assisted videokeratography was evaluated for improvement or worsening.[3] Both the videokeratoscope image and the computer-generated topography maps were examined for changes in corneal surface irregularity between the preoperative and final postoperative examinations. Subjective patient improvement was determined by both patient questionnaire and physician assessment at the time of the examination.

Results

LASER PULSES AND PACHYMETRY

The number of laser pulses ranged from 15 in patients with epithelial basement membrane dystrophy and recurrent erosion syndrome to 1,095 in a case of Reis-Buckler's dystrophy (Table 4–2). The average number of pulses applied was 418; the average was 643 in the general PTK group (n = 8), 498 in the superficial keratectomy group (n = 3), 36 in the epithelial basement

Table 4–2.   Study 1: Laser Pulses and Pachymetry

Treatment Group	Average No. of Laser Pulses	Average Decrease in Pachymetry (μm)
General PTK	643	46
Superficial keratectomy/PTK	498	110
Superficial scar removal	524	69
Focal PTK	296	36
Epithelial basement membrane Dystrophy/recurrent erosion	36	1

Source: Reprinted with permission from Hersh et al.[1] Courtesy of *Ophthalmology.*

membrane dystrophy group (n = 5), 524 in the superficial scar group (n = 5), and 296 in the focal treatment group (n = 7). Preoperative corneal thickness ranged from 470 to 704 µm, with a mean of 560 µm. Postoperative values ranged from 432 to 611 µm, with a mean of 529. An average of 31 µm of tissue was removed with the procedure in general; the average removed was 46 µm in the general PTK group (n = 8), 110 µm in the superficial keratectomy group (n = 3), 1 µm in the epithelial basement membrane dystrophy group (n = 5), 69 µm in the superficial scar group (n = 3), and 36 µm in the focal treatment group (n = 7).

VISUAL ACUITY

Preoperative and postoperative uncorrected and best-corrected visual acuities are summarized in Figures 4–1 and 4–2. Uncorrected visual acuity im-

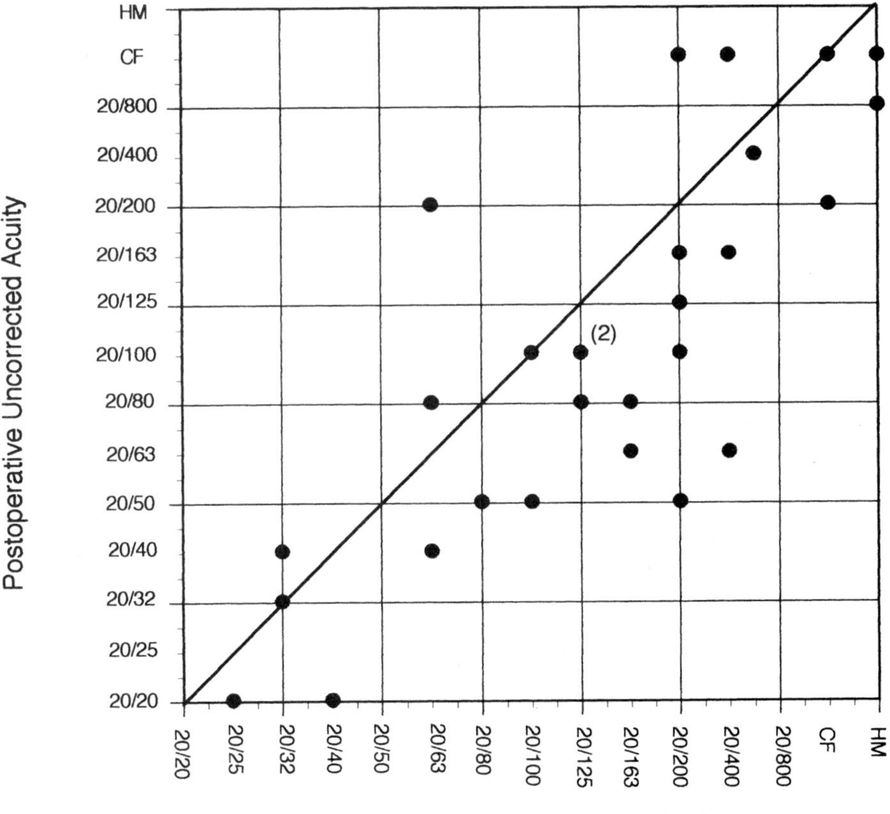

Figure 4–1.   Scattergram showing preoperative versus postoperative uncorrected visual acuity of individual patients. For points depicting more than one patient, the actual number is indicated above and to the right of the point. (Reproduced with permission from Hersh et al.[1] Courtesy of *Ophthalmology*.)

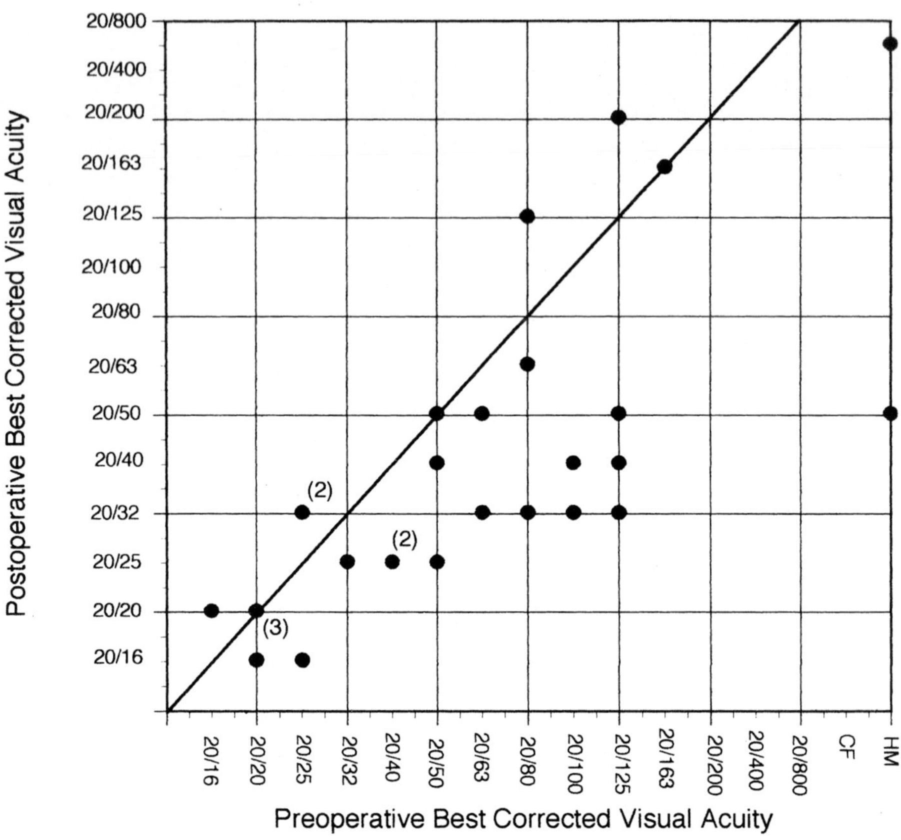

Figure 4–2. Scattergram showing preoperative versus postoperative best-corrected spectacle visual acuity of individual patients. For points depicting more than one patient, the actual number is indicated above and to the right of the point. (Reproduced with permission from Hersh et al.[1] Courtesy of *Ophthalmology*.)

proved in 20 eyes (with 14 improving 2 or more Snellen lines), remained unchanged in 3, and decreased in 5 (Fig. 4–3). Of those losing uncorrected visual acuity, two were in the general group, one had a superficial scar, one was in the epithelial basement membrane dystrophies group, and one had undergone combined superficial keratectomy and PTK. Spectacle-corrected visual acuity improved in 20 eyes (with 13 improving 2 or more lines), remained unchanged in 3, and decreased in 5 (Fig. 4–4). Two patients had 2 Snellen lines of best-corrected visual acuity loss. Of the two, one had an increase in cataract. The other was treated for a corneal stromal scar with consequent distortion in the postoperative corneal topography. Correction with a rigid gas-permeable contact lens, however, led to an increase in visual acuity of one line in this patient.

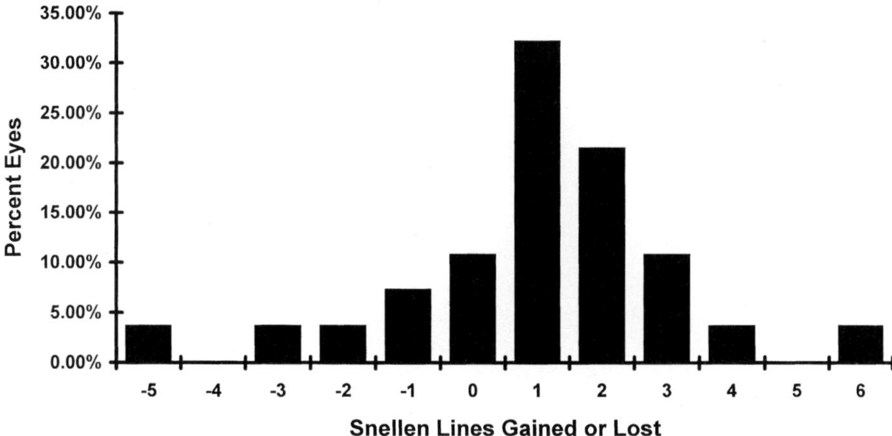

Figure 4–3.   Change in uncorrected visual acuity following PTK. (Reproduced with permission from Hersh et al.[1] Courtesy of *Ophthalmology*.)

ASTIGMATISM

Preoperative astigmatism ranged from 0 to 5.5 diopters, averaging 2.1 diopters, while postoperative astigmatism ranged from 0 to 5.5 diopters, averaging 2.0 diopters. Thus, although individuals showed variable changes in astigmatism with the procedure, when taken as a group there was little change in keratometric astigmatism with the PTK procedure.

PATIENTS' SUBJECTIVE ASSESSMENT

Nineteen patients (21 eyes) noted subjective improvement in their symptomatology, while seven reported no change. All patients with photophobia and ocular surface discomfort reported improvement. The one patient with a complaint of monocular multiplopia due to Salzmann's degeneration noted complete resolution of symptoms while four of five patients with recurrent epithelial erosive symptoms reported improvement. Twenty-one of the 26 patients reported that they would undergo the procedure again based on their initial experience.

Study 2

Study Design

In a prospective multicenter study[4] of the Summit OmniMed ExciMed excimer laser, 232 eyes of 211 patients were treated at 13 centers. Mean follow up was 10 ± 8 months. Eligible eyes had a corneal opacity in the anterior 100 µm of the corneal stroma or corneal surface irregularity. Eyes with a corneal thickness of less than 400 µm were excluded from the study. The goal

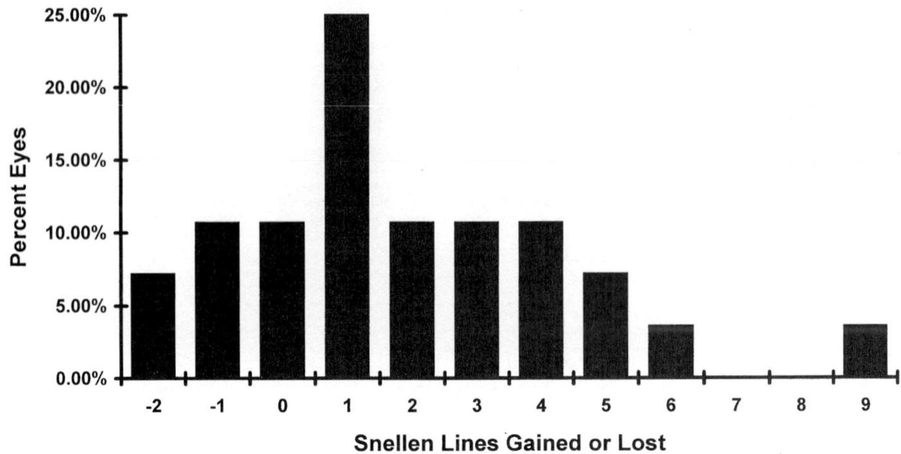

Figure 4–4.   Change in best-corrected spectacle visual acuity following PTK. (Reproduced with permission from Hersh et al.[1] Courtesy of *Ophthalmology*.)

of treatment in all cases was improvement in spectacle-corrected visual acuity. Laser parameters were the same as described in study 1.

Results

LASER PULSES

An average of 643 ± 1,003 pulses was used with a range of 15–10,742 pulses for each PTK treatment.

VISUAL ACUITY

At 1 year postoperatively, spectacle-corrected visual acuity improved in 46 (45%) of 103 eyes and worsened in 9 (9%) of 103 eyes by 2 or more Snellen lines. Spectacle corrrected visual acuity improved by a mean of 1.6 ± 2.8 Snellen lines, with a range of 12 lines gained to 5 lines lost. The mean improvement in Snellen lines of spectacle-corrected visual acuity was 0.1 for band keratopathy, 1.1 for epithelial basement membrane dystrophy, 1.2 for corneal scars, 1.6 for Salzmann's nodular degeneration, and 2.4 for corneal dystrophies.

ASTIGMATISM

Of 87 eyes at 1 year follow up, the average astigmatism decreased by 0.36 diopters. Seventeen eyes (20%) had an increase of 1.0 diopter or more of astigmatism while 19 (22%) had a decrease of 1.0 diopter or more. The largest increase in astigmatism was 4.50 diopters, and the largest decrease was 10.50 diopters.

Conclusions

When defining improvement in spectacle-corrected visual acuity as the goal of treatment, PTK was most effective in the treatment of corneal dystrophies, Salzmann's nodular degeneration, and corneal scars. PTK was least effective in the treatment of calcific band keratopathy.

Study 3

Study Design

In a single center study[5] using the VisX Twenty-Twenty excimer laser (VisX Corporation, Sunnyvale, CA), 18 eyes with corneal opacities were treated. Patients were divided into four categories: corneal dystrophies, corneal scars secondary to previous infectious corneal ulcers, scars secondary to trauma, and calcific band keratopathy. Laser parameters included a fluence of 160 mJ/cm^2 and a repetition rate of 5 Hz. In these cases, the laser was set to perform a direct ablation (without "polishing") of a thickness determined by preoperative measurement of the corneal scar using optical pachymetry.

Results

Spectacle-corrected visual acuity improved in 9 patients (50.0%), remained unchanged in 6 patients (33.3%), and decreased in 3 patients (16.7%). Three patients had improvement of visual acuity with rigid gas-permeable contact lenses compared with visual acuity achieved with spectacles. Uncorrected visual acuity improved in all patients with corneal dystrophies and in approximately half of eyes with corneal scars. No improvement in vision was seen in those patients with calcific band keratopathy.

Study 4

One large study[6] of climatic droplet keratopathy performed by one of the authors (MDW) affords the opportunity to examine the results of a large, prospective series of a single corneal disorder and presents a unique opportunity to subject important parameters of outcome and potential complications to statistical analysis. Comparison of the results for smooth climatic droplet keratopathy, where the pathology is largely confined to Bowman's layer, with that of irregular climatic droplet keratopathy, where there is extension into the anterior stroma, also provides an opportunity to study outcomes in eyes at both ends of the spectrum of technical difficulty. Furthermore, in contrast to the aforementioned investigations, analysis of the risk of complications for a single disorder with a well-defined spectrum of associated ocular surface disease (smooth = relatively mild, irregular = moderately severe) allows evaluation of the contribution of the severity of pre-existing ocular surface disease to complication rates in PTK.

While climatic droplet keratopathy is not of great clinical significance in Western countries,[7-9] it is a major source of visual disability in regions such as Saudi Arabia, where the prevalence of blindness related to corneal scarring from climatic droplet keratopathy and other disorders is very high (17.3% of all cases of blindness).[10] The complication rates associated with lamellar or penetrating keratoplasty in this region are high,[11] making the development of less risky alternative therapy such as PTK an important clinical advance.

In this study of one specific disease process, PTK was found to be very successful in reducing corneal opacification and improving uncorrected and best-corrected visual acuity in eyes with climatic droplet keratopathy.[6] In eyes with combined cataract and climatic droplet keratopathy, treatment was also found to be effective in improving visualization and facilitating subsequent cataract extraction, eliminating the necessity for performing riskier combined penetrating keratoplasty and cataract extraction.[6]

Results

CORNEAL CLARITY

In this study,[6] corneal clarity after PTK was graded as clear/trace, mild, moderate, and severe. The final corneal clarity was mild or better in 54/55 (98%) eyes with smooth climatic droplet keratopathy (Fig. 4–5, Case 14) compared with 16/20 (80%) in eyes with irregular climatic droplet keratopathy ($p = 0.00003$; Table 4–3).

VISUAL ACUITY

Eyes with smooth climatic droplet keratopathy were more likely to obtain more than one line of improved uncorrected (56% vs. 25%) or spectacle-corrected visual acuity (61.8% vs. 21.2%) than those with irregular climatic droplet keratopathy ($p = 0.03$ and 0.005, respectively); (Tables 4–4, 4–5). There was not a significant difference between the two groups in the incidence of loss of uncorrected or spectacle-corrected visual acuity (defined as more than 1 line of Snellen acuity). In many cases, failure to improve or worsening was related to progressive cataract formation. In three cases (two irregular, one smooth) worsening of vision postoperatively was due to microbial keratitis-induced scarring.

DELAYED RE-EPITHELIALIZATION/SECONDARY MICROBIAL KERATITIS

There was an increase in delayed re-epithelialization (> 14 days) in eyes with irregular climatic droplet keratopathy (21%) compared with eyes with smooth climatic droplet keratopathy (9%) following PTK. This complication

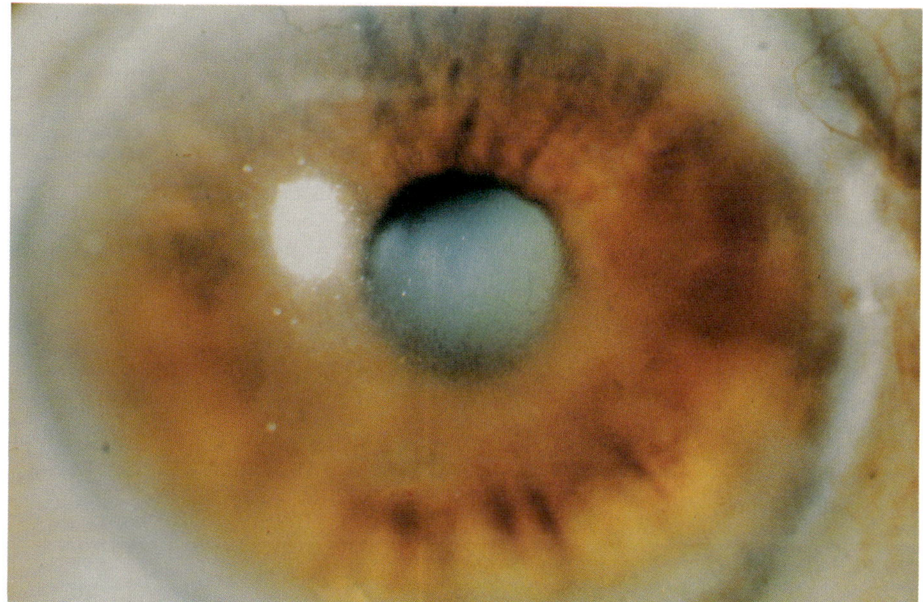

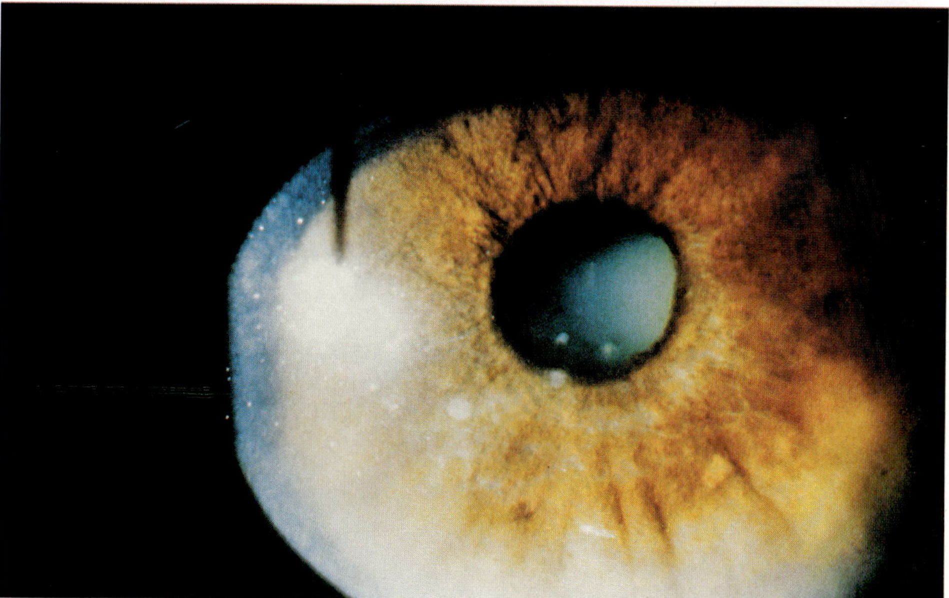

Figure 4–5.   Case 14. Smooth climatic droplet keratopathy. **(A)** Preoperative. There is central corneal opacification at the level of Bowman's layer with obscuration of iris details. **(B)** Postoperative appearance. The reduction in corneal opacification, improved clarity of iris details, and improved visualization of a significant cataract is obvious. There was no change in visual acuity until after subsequent cataract extraction. (Reproduced with permission from Badr et al.[6])

Table 4–3.   Study 4: Corneal Clarity After Phototherapeutic Keratectomy for Climatic Droplet Keratopathy (CDK)

GRADE	SMOOTH CDK	IRREGULAR CDK	OVERALL
Clear/trace	44/55 (80%)*	5/20 (25%)*	49/75 (65.33%)
Mild	10/55 (18%)	11/20 (55%)	21/75 (28.00%)
Moderate	1/55 (2%)	3/20 (15%)	4/75 (5.33%)
Severe	0	1/20 (5%)	1/75 (1.33%)

* Significant difference between smooth/irregular, $p = 0.00003$.
CDK, climatic droplet keratopathy.
Reproduced with permission from Badr et al.[6]

Table 4–4.   Study 4: Change in Uncorrected Visual Acuity After Phototherapeutic Keratectomy for Climatic Droplet Keratopathy (CDK)

CHANGE	SMOOTH CDK	IRREGULAR CDK	OVERALL
Improved (>1 line)	31/55 (56.4%)*	5/20 (25.0%)*	36/75 (48.0%)
No change (±1 line)	20/55 (36.4%)	13/20 (65.0%)	33/75 (44.0%)
Decreased (>1 line)	4/55 (7.2%)	2/20 (10.0%)	6/75 (8.0%)

* Significant difference between smooth/irregular, $p = 0.03$.
CDK, climatic droplet keratopathy.
Reproduced with permission from Badr et al.[6]

Table 4–5.   Study 4: Change in Spectacle-Corrected Visual Acuity After Phototherapeutic Keratectomy for Climatic Droplet Keratopathy (CDK)

CHANGE	SMOOTH CDK	IRREGULAR CDK	OVERALL
Improved (>1 line)	34/55 (61.8%)*	4/18 (22.2%)*	38/73 (52.1%)
No change (±1 line)	15/55 (27.3%)	11/18 (61.1%)	26/73 (35.6%)
Decreased (>1 line)	6/55 (10.9%)	3/18 (16.7%)	9/73 (12.3%)
Not available		1	1

* Significant difference between smooth/irregular, $p = 0.005$.
CDK, climatic droplet keratopathy.
Reproduced with permission from Badr et al.[6]

correlated with the increased incidence of secondary microbial keratitis (10% vs. 1.8%) in the eyes with irregular climatic droplet keratopathy.[12]

KERATOMETRIC CHANGES

There was an average flattening of the corneal curvature from a preoperative average of 43.1 (standard deviation = 2.1) diopters, to 41.3 (3.1) diopters at 3 months, 40.7 (2.4) diopters at 6 months, and 41.8 (4.0) diopters at 12 months. There was statistically significant postoperative flattening of the cornea ($p <$ 0.05) when compared with preoperative measurements (see Chapter 6).

There was not a statistically significant change in keratometric readings at 6 months or 1 year compared with the measurements at 3 months.

Conclusions

One of the most striking results in this study[6] was consistently superior corneal clarity and visual acuity when comparing smooth climatic droplet keratopathy to irregular climatic droplet keratopathy. This difference can be accounted for by the more advanced state of irregular climatic droplet keratopathy, where there has been extension into the anterior stroma, thereby making PTK technically more difficult. The molecular weight of the climatic droplet keratopathy globules has been shown to be 67,000,[13] which differs considerably from the collagen stromal matrix. It is reasonable to assume that different ablation rates of the pathology and the normal collagen stroma will occur. As a result, even the most diligent use of masking fluids[14,15] will not ensure a completely even ablation, especially in cases of irregular climatic droplet keratopathy, resulting in retention of some of the preoperative variable corneal thickness and irregular astigmatism (Figs. 3–16; 4–6, Case 15).

The irregular extension of the disease process into the anterior stroma in irregular climatic droplet keratopathy makes complete elimination of the scar more difficult than with smooth climatic droplet keratopathy, where the pathology is entirely at the level of Bowman's layer (Fig, 4–5, Case 14). The more advanced pre-existing ocular surface abnormalities in irregular climatic droplet keratopathy is well known,[16] and it is therefore not surprising that these eyes have a higher incidence of delayed re-epithelialization[6] and secondary microbial keratitis following PTK.[12]

Other Studies of Specific Corneal Disorders

Although recurrent epithelial erosions secondary to epithelial basement membrane dystrophy and other dystrophies and degenerations can be treated with the PTK procedure, recurrent erosion syndrome per se is not an indication approved by the FDA. However, in one study of 74 eyes using the MEL 50 Aesculap-Meditec excimer laser,[17] 55 (74%) eyes were recurrence free.

Although keratoconus is a contraindication for excimer laser refractive treatment, success has been reported in the treatment of raised nodular scars causing pain and contact lens intolerance in keratoconus patients.[18] Investigators have reported success with such treatments in four cases.[19]

In a study of three eyes with trachoma-induced corneal scarring,[20] investigators have shown successful visual recovery. One patient had a refractive hyperopic shift of +9 diopters, however.

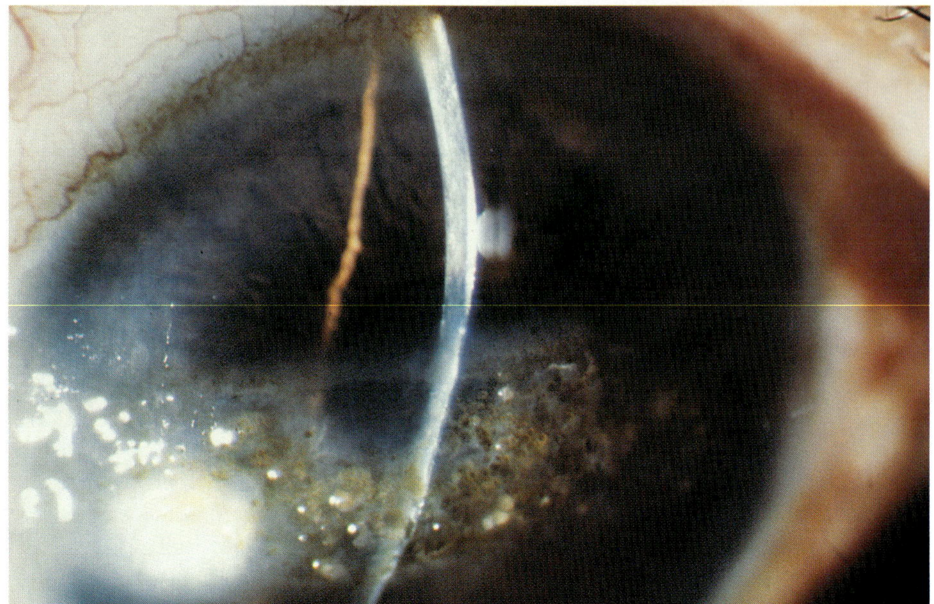

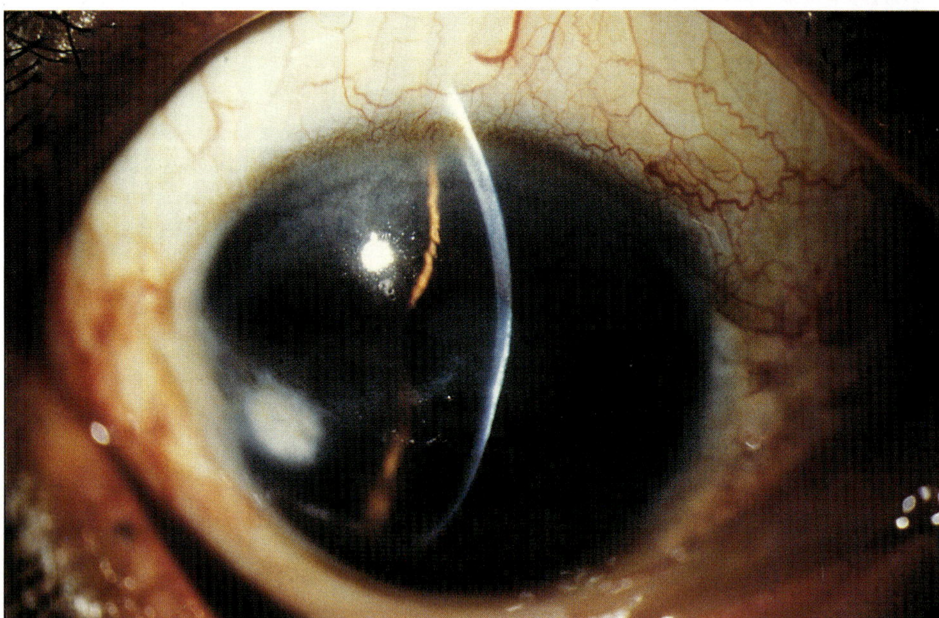

Figure 4–6. Case 15. Irregular climatic droplet keratopathy. **(A)** Preoperative. Golden-yellow globular deposits are present in a band-shaped configuration in the visual axis with marked irregularity of the surface and extension of corneal opacification into the anterior stroma. **(B)** Postoperative. After manually scraping the globular deposits and excimer ablation of Bowman's layer and anterior stroma, the corneal clarity is improved, but corneal thinning, mild scarring, and some irregularity still persists. Visual acuity improved from CF 4 feet to 20/200. (Reproduced with permission from Badr et al.[6])

One case has been reported in which recurrent corneal intraepithelial dysplasia was successfully treated.[26] A clear cornea was maintained for a 26 month follow-up period, with improvement in visual acuity from hand motions to 20/100. Similarly, conjunctival epithelial melanosis has also been reported as amenable to treatment with PTK.[22]

Conclusions

As is evident, results of PTK may vary considerably depending on the goal of treatment and the type of disorder treated. Even individuals with a similar disease process may have variable treatment results depending on the severity of the disease.

References

1. Hersh PS, Burnstein Y, Carr J, Etwaru G, Mayers M. Phototherapeutic keratectomy: surgical strategies and clinical outcomes. Ophthalmology 1996;103:1210–1222.
2. Holladay JT, Prager TC. Mean visual acuity [letter]. Am J Ophthalmol 1991;111:372–374.
3. Hersh PS, Schwartz-Goldstein B. Summit PRK Topography Study Group. Corneal topography of phase III excimer laser photorefractive keratectomy: characterization and clinical effects. Ophthalmology 1995;102:963–978.
4. Maloney RK, Thompson V, Ghiselli G, Durrie D, Waring GO, O'Connell M. A prospective multicenter trial of excimer laser phototherapeutic keratectomy for corneal vision loss. Am J Ophthalmol 1996;122:149–160.
5. Campos M, Nielson S, Szerenyi K, Garbus JJ, McDonnell PJ. Clinical followup of phototherapeutic keratectomy for treatment of corneal opacities. Am J Ophthalmol 1993;115:433–440.
6. Badr IA, Al-Rajhi A, Wagoner MD et al. Phototherapeutic keratectomy for climatic droplet keratopathy. J Refract Surg 1996;12:114–122.
7. Gray RH, Johnson GJ, Freedman A. Climatic droplet keratopathy. Surv Ophthalmol 1992;36:241–253.
8. Freedman A. Climatic droplet keratopathy. I. Clinical aspects. Arch Ophthalmol 1973;89:193–197.
9. Tabbara KF. Climatic droplet keratopathy. Int Ophthalmol Clin 1986;26:63–68.
10. Badr IA, Al-Saif AM, Al-Rajhi AA, Cavender JC et al. Changing patterns of visual loss in the Eastern Province, Kingdom of Saudi Arabia. Saudi J Ophthalmol 1992;6:59–68.
11. Hazzaa SA, Tabbara KF. Bacterial keratitis after penetrating keratoplasty. Ophthalmology 1988;95:1504–1508.
12. Al-Rajhi AA, Wagoner MD, Badr IA, Saif A, Mahmood M. Bacterial keratitis following phototherapeutic keratectomy. J Refract Surg 1996;12:123–127.
13. Duhaiman AS, Aprahamian S, Gorban AM, Shourkey N, Tabbara K. Biochemical analysis of climatic droplet keratopathy. Saudi Bull Ophthalmol 1988;3:147–149.
14. McDonnell JM, Garbus JJ, McDonnell PJ. Unsuccessful excimer laser PTK. Clinicopathologic correlation. Arch Ophthalmol 1992;110:977–979.
15. Kornmehl E, Steinert RF, Puliafito CA. A comparative study of masking fluids for excimer laser PTK. Arch Ophthalmol 1991;109:860–863.
16. Ormerod DL, Dahan E, Hagele JE, Guzek JP. Serious occurrences in the natural history of advanced climatic keratopathy. Ophthalmology 1994;101:448–453.
17. Dausch D, Landesz M, Klein R, Schroder E. Phototherapeutic keratectomy in recurrent epithelial erosion. J Refract Corneal Surg 1993;9:419–424.
18. Steinert RF, Puliafito CA. Excimer laser phototherapeutic keratectomy for a corneal nodule. Refract Corneal Surg 1990;6:352.
19. Ward MA, Artunduaga G, Thompson KP, Wilson LA, Stulting RD. Phototherapeutic keratectomy frot the treatment of nodular subepithelial corneal scars in patients with keratoconus who are contact lens intolerant. CLAO J 1995;21:130–132.

20. Goldstein M, Loewenstein A, Rosner M, Lipshitz I, Lazar M. Phototherapeutic keratectomy in the treatment of corneal scarring from trachoma. J Refract Corneal Surg 1994;10:S290–S292.
21. Dausch D, Landesz M, Schroder E. Phototherapeutic keratectomy in recurrent corneal intraepithelial dysplasia. Arch Ophthalmol 1994;112:22–23.
22. Kim JH, Hahn TW. Excimer laser ablation of conjunctival epithelial melanosis. J Cataract Refract Surg 1993;19:309–311.

5

Complications

In contrast to excimer laser photorefractive keratectomy, which is performed on healthy eyes, the laser in PTK is a surgical tool that is generally used on diseased corneas. Therefore, complications associated with corneal surgery in general may apply to PTK. In addition, topography and refractive changes may cause additional side effects of PTK in particular.

There are three postoperative healing stages following PTK. Re-epithelialization takes from a few days to weeks in some patients. Stromal remodeling occurs over the succeeding weeks and months, while topography and refractive changes may take months to stabilize. Consequently, general postoperative goals include encouragement of epithelialization, minimization of stromal scarring, and the optimization of refractive and topography results (Fig. 5–1).

Specific Complications

Epithelialization Problems

Many patients undergoing PTK suffer previous ocular surface disease. Loss of epithelial vitality may lead to problems with epithelialization following the procedure (Fig. 5–2). Particularly in patients with damage to the limbal stem cell population, which is necessary to support a clear and lustrous epithelial surface, subsequent epithelialization may be problematic, and sterile corneal ulceration may supervene. Patients, therefore, should be properly selected for the procedure. Those with severe ocular surface disease such as chemical burns, ocular cicatricial pemphigoid, atopic keratoconjunctivitis, and severe keratitis sicca should be treated with caution. In such patients, autologous or heterologous limbal conjunctival transplantation may be the procedure of choice.[1]

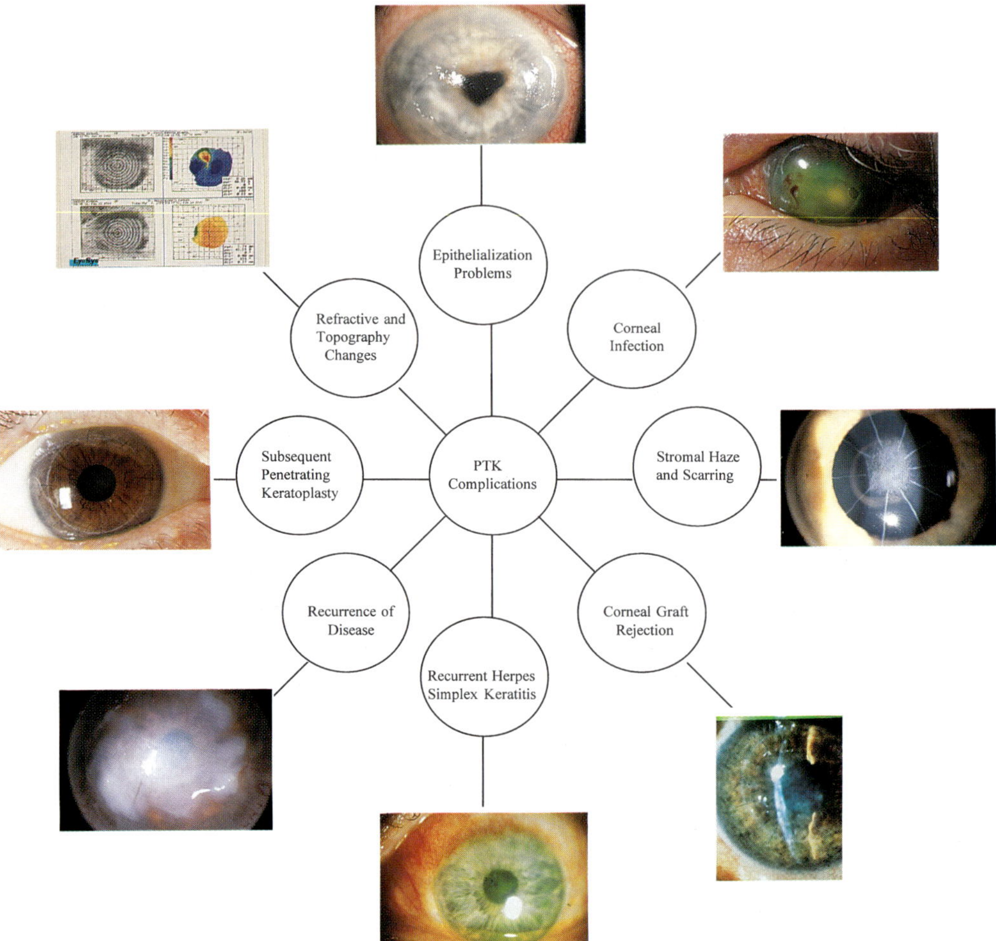

Figure 5–1.   Schematic of PTK complications.

In the face of persistent epithelial defects or recurrent epithelial breakdown, efforts should be made to promote epithelialization. These include lubrication, preferably with nonpreserved solutions and ointments. In addition, a bandage soft contact lens may support and protect the epithelium during the healing process. Careful examination should identify lid problems such as malposition and blepharitis, which may be precipitating or adding to problems with epithelialization. An inflamed ocular surface may diminish epithelialization, and judicious use of corticosteroids may be helpful. In addition, modification of the ocular surface environment with tetracylcine derivatives may benefit patients with meibomitis or a sterile corneal ulceration. In rare cases, temporary tarsorrhaphy may be helpful.

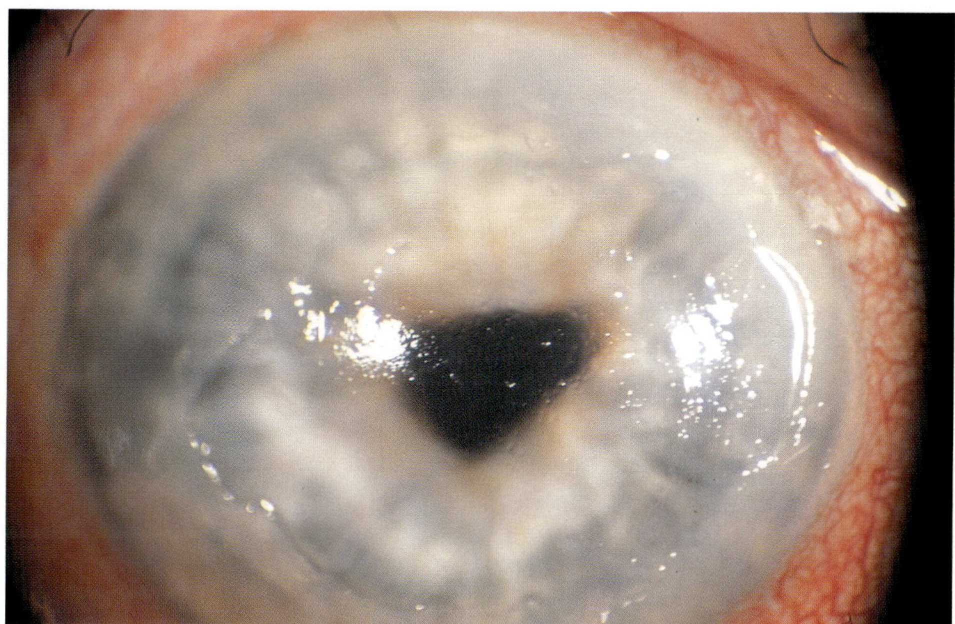

Figure 5–2.   Persistent epithelial defect following PTK for a corneal scar secondary to a toxic reaction.

In one study of 28 eyes,[2] epithelial healing occurred within 3 days in 19 eyes and between 3 days and 1 week in 6 eyes. One patient with Salzmann's degeneration, one with a corneal scar and preoperative epitheliopathy, and one patient with contact lens induced keratopathy required adjunctive use of a bandage soft contact lens and up to 1 month for complete re-epithelialization. The patient with a contact lens related keratopathy required a bandage soft contact lens to promote complete healing and had a recurrence of an optically poor epithelial surface despite initially successful PTK (Fig. 5–3, Case 16).

In a study of 18 eyes using the VisX excimer laser, no eyes had re-epithelialization difficulty or problems with subsequent epithelial dysadherence.In another study, a large, prospective series of eyes with climatic droplet ker-

Figure 5–3. *(Following two pages)*   Case 16. **(A)** Soft contact lens keratopathy preoperatively in a 34-year-old woman. **(B)** Cleared cornea following PTK with increased comfort and improved visual acuity. **(C)** Videokeratoscope image before **(Top Left)** and 1 month after **(Bottom Left)** PTK showing a marked improvement in corneal surface regularity. The corresponding computerized topographic maps **(Right)** demonstrate smooth and symmetrical corneal flattening. **(D)** Reaccumulation of abnormal epithelium 3 months postoperatively.

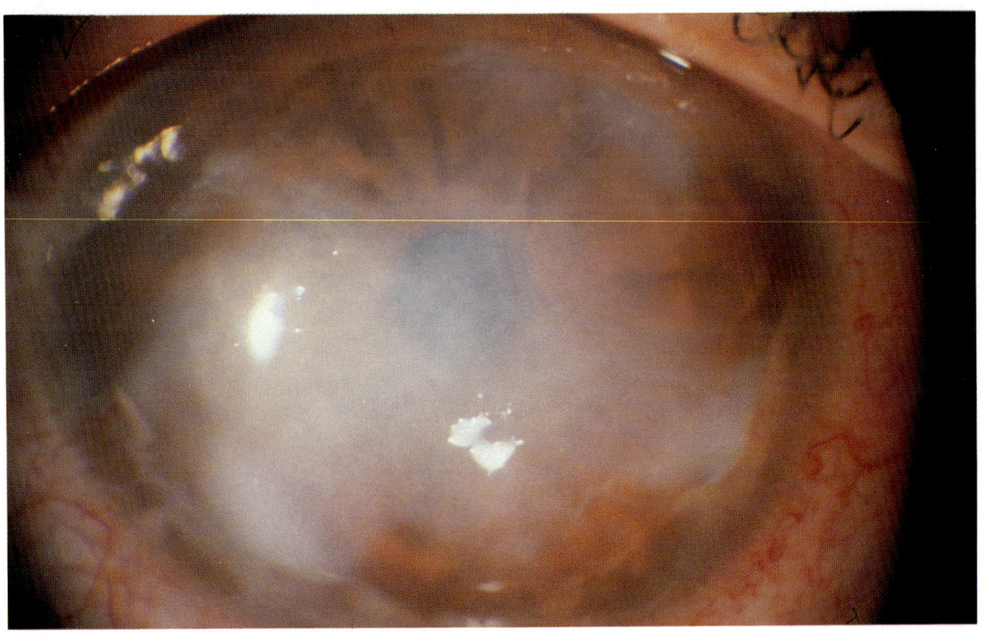

Figure 5–3 (A)

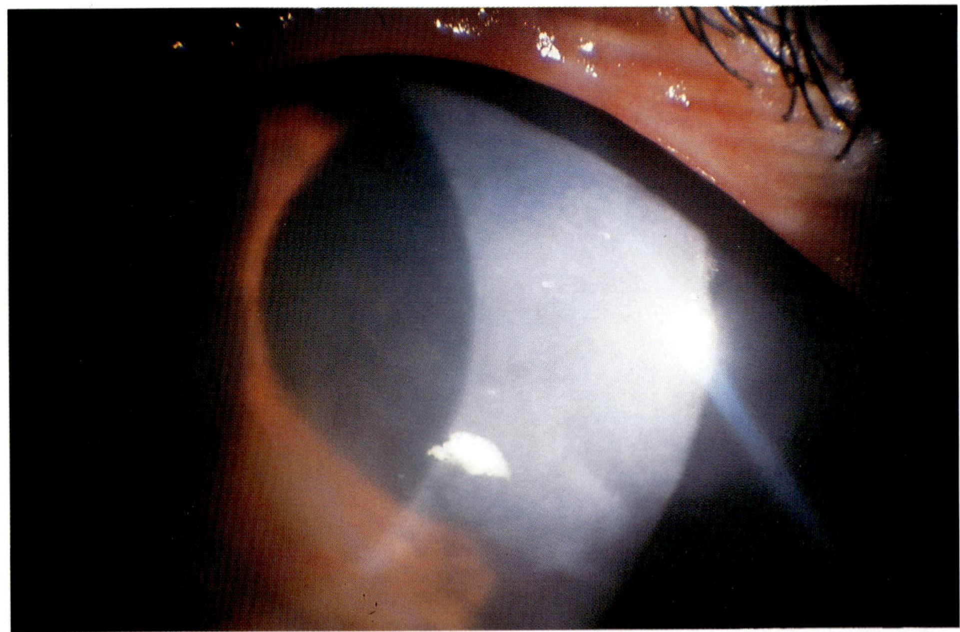

Figure 5–3 (B)

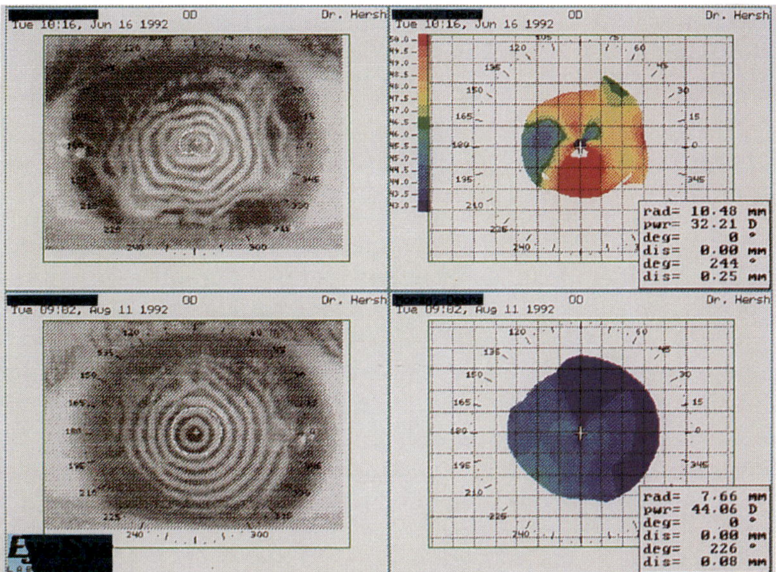

Figure 5–3 (C)

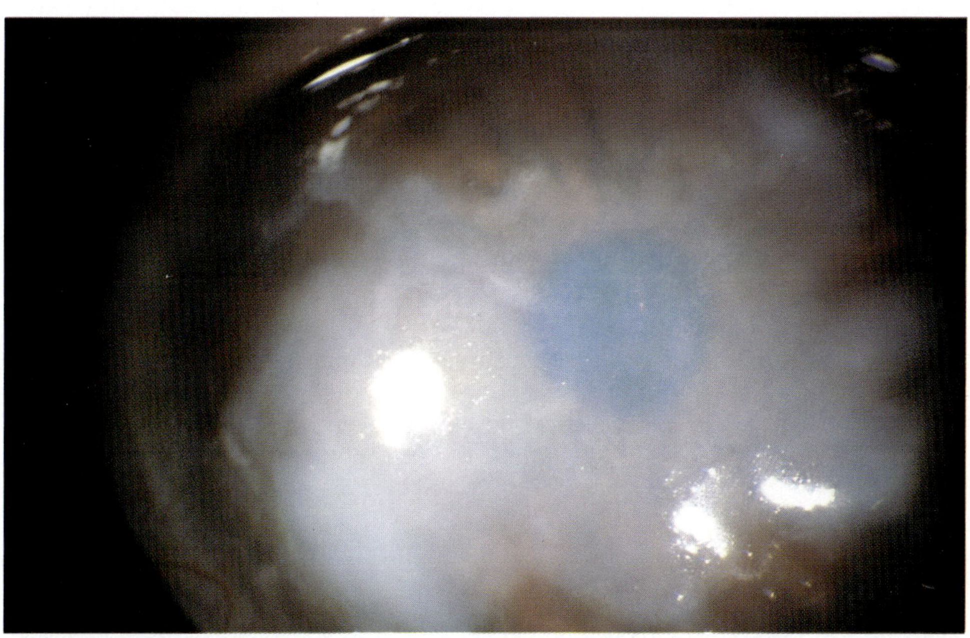

Figure 5–3 (D)

atopathy treated with PTK were analyzed.[3] In these patients, delayed re-epithelialization (>14 days) was the most frequent complication, occurring in 12% of eyes treated.

Corneal Infection

The risk of microbial keratitis due to the iatrogenic introduction of an epithelial defect following treatment of superficial corneal disorders with either manual or phototherapeutic keratectomy is low,[4] but this is a serious complication that can adversely affect the final visual outcome. The greatest risk of microbial keratitis following PTK is either before re-epithelialization is complete or within the first few weeks after re-epithelialization before the risk of recurrent epithelial erosion is virtually eliminated.[3,5] Moreover, the previously diseased cornea is at greater risk of infection following surgery than the healthy cornea. Persistent epithelial defects in such eyes may afford an inviting substrate for microbial keratitis. Thus, infection will be discouraged with prompt re-epithelialization of the defect and strenuous efforts should be made to avoid persistent epithelial defects. In addition, antibiotic prophylactics with a nontoxic antibiotic (such as a fluroquinolone) is suggested. Following PTK, the patient should be closely followed in the face of a persistent epithelial defect especially if a bandage soft contact lens is in place.[6] Any infiltrates should be promptly cultured and infections treated with broad-spectrum antibiotic coverage.

In a large series of 166 eyes undergoing PTK, Fagerholm et al.[7] did not specifically address the issue of the incidence of postoperative microbial keratitis, although the discussion implies that no cases of microbial keratitis were seen postoperatively. In another study of 232 eyes,[8] one eye developed bacterial keratitis and one patient developed marginal corneal ulceration thought to be secondary to systemic vasculitis. A Wessely-type immune ring has also been reported following PTK.[9]

To date, only one large, prospective clinical trial has specifically addressed the incidence of microbial keratitis following PTK. Microbial keratitis was reported in three (1.2%) of 258 consecutive eyes undergoing PTK in Saudi Arabia.[5] In this study, all three cases of microbial keratitis were in 183 eyes (1.6%) with a diagnosis of climatic droplet keratopathy, while no cases were observed in 75 eyes with other anterior corneal disorders (corneal scarring, Salzmann's nodular degeneration, granular dystrophy, band keratopathy, and vernal shield ulcers). There was a marked increase in secondary microbial keratitis in eyes with irregular (10.0%) versus smooth (1.8%) climatic droplet keratopathy, a finding consistent with more severe pre-existing ocular surface abnormalities[10] and an increased incidence of delayed re-epithelialization postoperatively.[3] Gram-positive species (*Streptococcus pneumonia* in two, coagulase-negative *Staphylococcus* in one) were the predominant species isolated from all three cases, a finding consistent with microbial keratitis seen in similar patient populations undergoing penetrating keratoplasty.[11–15] In two cases, the microbial keratitis was associated with delayed re-epithelialization, occurring 21 and 73 days (Fig. 5–4, Case 17) postoperatively. In the third case, microbial keratitis appeared 16 days after re-epithelialization was complete due to a recurrent epithelial erosion (Fig. 5–5, Case 18). In all three cases the visual outcome was adversely affected, with the final visual acuity ranging from 20/125 to 20/400.

The overall risk of bacterial keratitis was small following PTK in this study and favorably compares with the risks of microbial keratitis following more invasive procedures such as lamellar and penetrating keratoplasty.[11–15] It is well established that not only are epithelial erosions and persistent epithelial defects rare following PTK, but that epithelial adhesion is actually improved following PTK, an observation that has led to its use in the treatment of recurrent erosions not amenable to conventional therapy.[10] Therefore, in the case of PTK for irregular climatic droplet keratopathy, not only is visual function often improved,[3] but it is possible that the improved epithelial adhesion may contribute to an actual reduction in the risk of microbial keratitis over the patient's lifetime.

Stromal Haze and Scarring

In general, excimer laser PTK has as one of its primary goals the amelioration of corneal opacity. Thus, postoperative stromal haze is of less concern for PTK than for PRK. Efforts promoting prompt epithelialization should mitigate an adverse stromal wound healing response. In addition, adjunctive use of topical corticosteroids may also be helpful in avoiding excessive keratocyte activation and scar formation.

In one study,[2] a trace to mild reticular subepithelial stromal haze was found in the treated area site of some patients. No eyes developed more than mild haze, and no frank scar formation was seen. In no case was the degree of haze or scar judged clinically significant.

Another investigation[8] found that the mean haze grade of 99 eyes preoperatively was 2.4 (scale = 0–4). At 6 months postoperatively, mean haze grade was 1.0, and at 1 year mean haze grade was 1.6. In 69 patients with preoperative haze, haze improved in 56 (81%) and worsened in 2 (3%).

Corneal Graft Reaction

There have been cases of immunological corneal graft reaction reported in the literature.[16,17] In one case, a 41-year-old woman with lattice corneal dystrophy had previously undergone successful penetrating keratoplasty.[17] Six years later, best-corrected visual acuity in the left eye had decreased from 20/25 to 20/80 because of recurrent lattice in the graft. Lattice deposits were seen beneath the epithelium and in the superficial corneal stroma (Fig. 5–6, Case 19). Computerized corneal topographic analysis demonstrated marked surface irregularity.

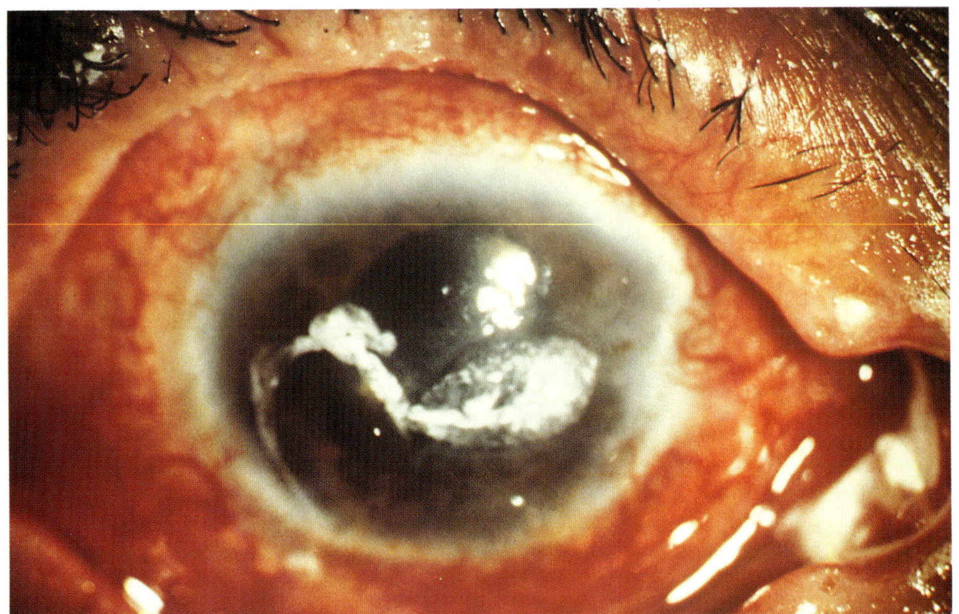

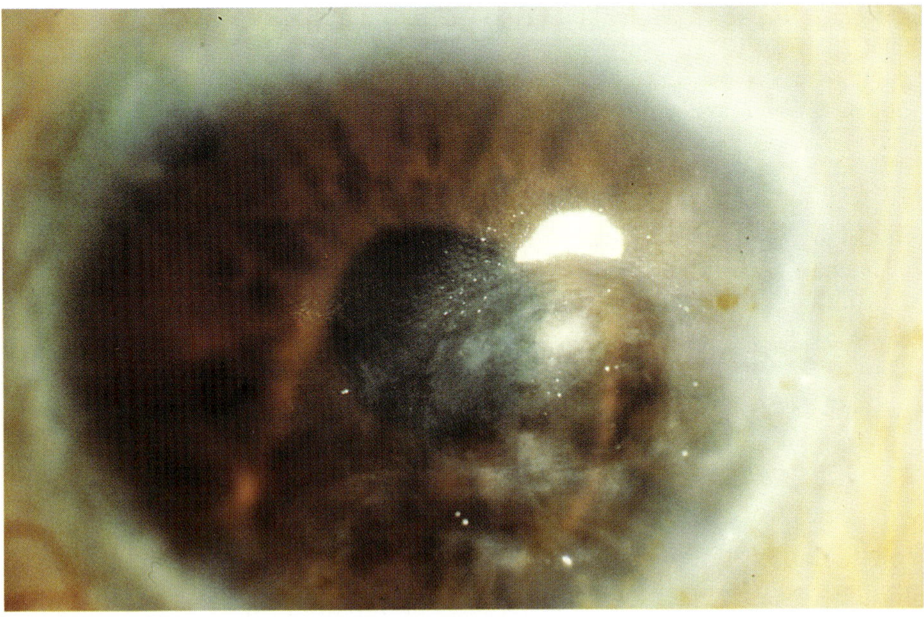

Figure 5–4.   Case 17. A 70-year-old Saudi male with irregular climatic droplet keratopathy. **(A)** Seventy-three days after phototherapeutic keratectomy, he presented with corneal infiltrate and positive cultures for coagulase-negative *Staphylococcus*. **(B)** Following resolution of the bacterial keratitis, persistent paracentral corneal thinning and scarring resulted in a final visual acuity of 20/400.

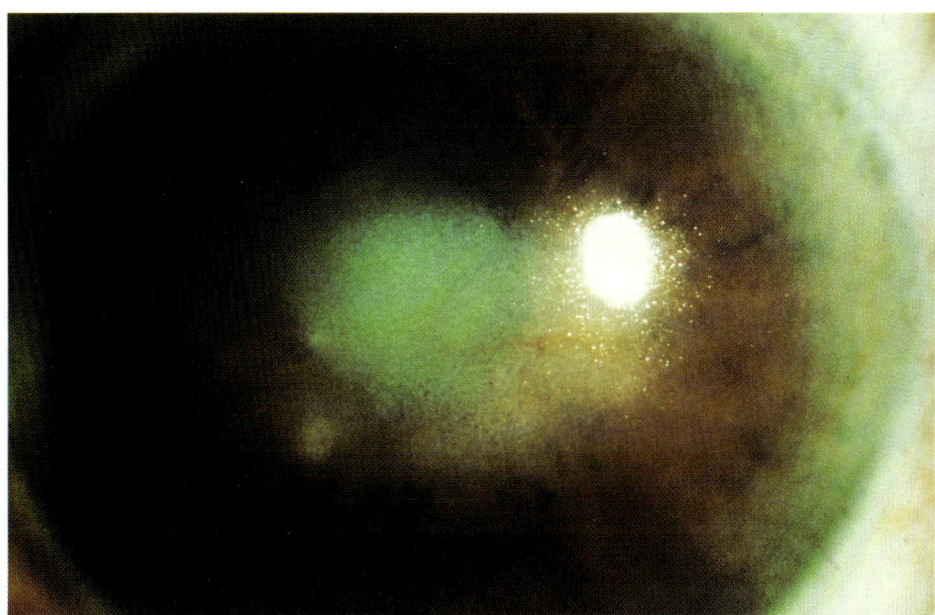

Figure 5–5. Case 18. **(A)** A 72-year-old Saudi male with smooth climatic droplet keratopathy and visual acuity of 20/100. *(Continued on following page)*

In treating the patient with the PTK procedure, after removing the epithelium overlying the area to be treated, methylcellulose 1% was applied to fill in surface irregularities. To optimize corneal smoothing, a polishing technique was used; the patient maintained fixation on the laser's fixation light while the eye was gently rotated by moving the patient's head as the procedure progressed. The patient was frequently examined at the slit lamp to determine areas to be further treated and to monitor the progress of the procedure. A total of 108 laser pulses were used. Postoperatively, the eye was patched, and tobramycin/dexamethasone ointment was applied five times daily.

One week postoperatively, uncorrected visual acuity had improved to 20/25. The corneal graft appeared much clearer and the stromal surface smoother. Since the epithelium remained somewhat irregular, however, a bandage soft contact lens was placed on the eye. One week later, the patient complained of decreased visual acuity and discomfort. On examination, visual acuity was 20/200 and the eye was inflamed, exhibiting an acute corneal rejection episode with moderate graft edema, keratic precipitates, and an endothelial rejection line (Fig. 5–6, Case 19). The patient was treated with prednisolone acetate 1% drops hourly, oral prednisone 80 mg daily, and subconjuctival triamcinolone 40 mg. Two weeks later, best-corrected visual acuity had returned to 20/25, the eye was uninflamed, and the corneal graft had

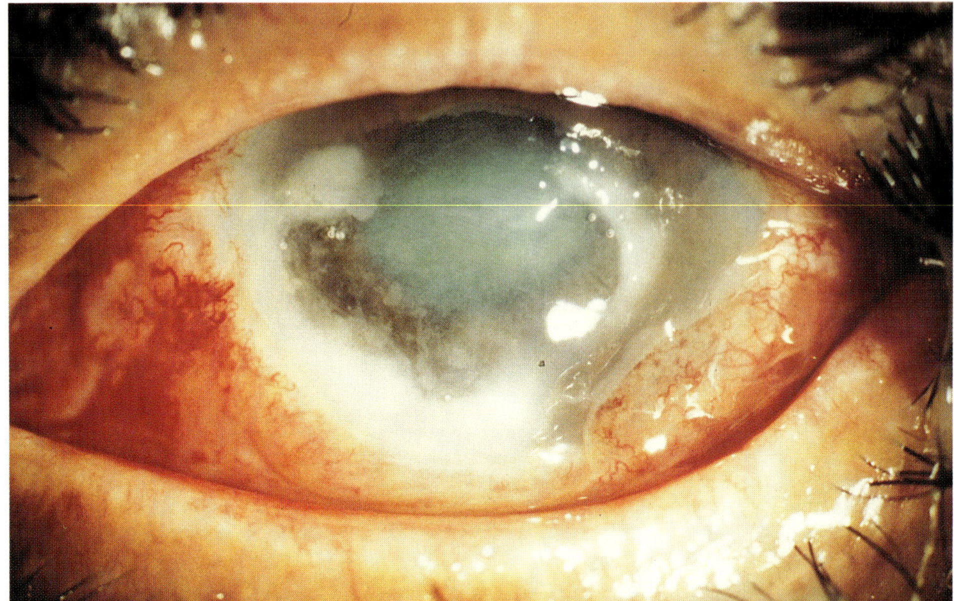

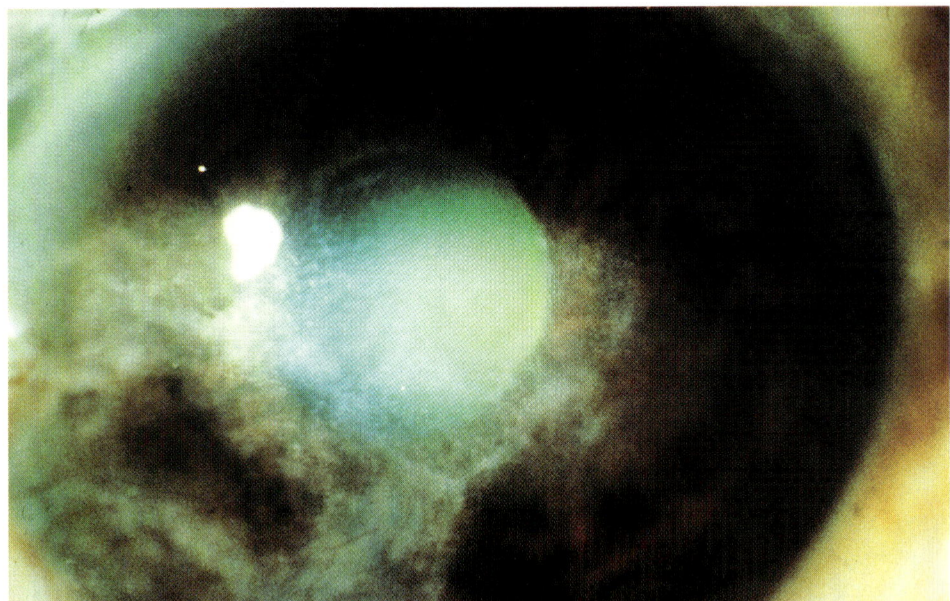

Figure 5–5 (B).   Twenty days postoperatively and 16 days after initial re-epithelialization, he presented with corneal infiltrate and positive cultures for *Streptococcus pneumonia.* **(C)** Following resolution of bacterial keratitis and after cataract extraction, persistent corneal scarring limited the final visual acuity to 20/125. (Reproduced by permission from Al-Rajhi et al.[5])

cleared without any residua of the rejection episode and has since remained stable. One additional case of an immunologic corneal graft reaction has been reported to date in the literature.[16]

Immunological corneal graft rejection has been reported years after penetrating keratoplasty and following minor manipulations to the cornea such as suture removal. It is thus unclear whether the episodes reported had been precipitated by the laser treatment itself, manual epithelial removal, bandage soft contact lens placement, or alterations in the patients' medical regimen. In all cases, corneal graft reactions should be promptly recognized and appropriately treated with corticosteroids.

Recurrent Herpes Simplex Keratitis

Reactivation of herpes simplex has been reported following PTK (Fig. 5–7, Case 20).[17, 18] In one large study of 232 eyes,[8] 3 eyes had recurrences of herpetic keratitis. As for corneal graft reactions, the etiology is unclear. The excimer laser emits light in the ultraviolet-C range, and there is also a visible blue fluorescence. These may account for some episodes of recurrence. In addition, manual trauma as well as postoperative use of corticosteroids may be factors in herpes reactivation.

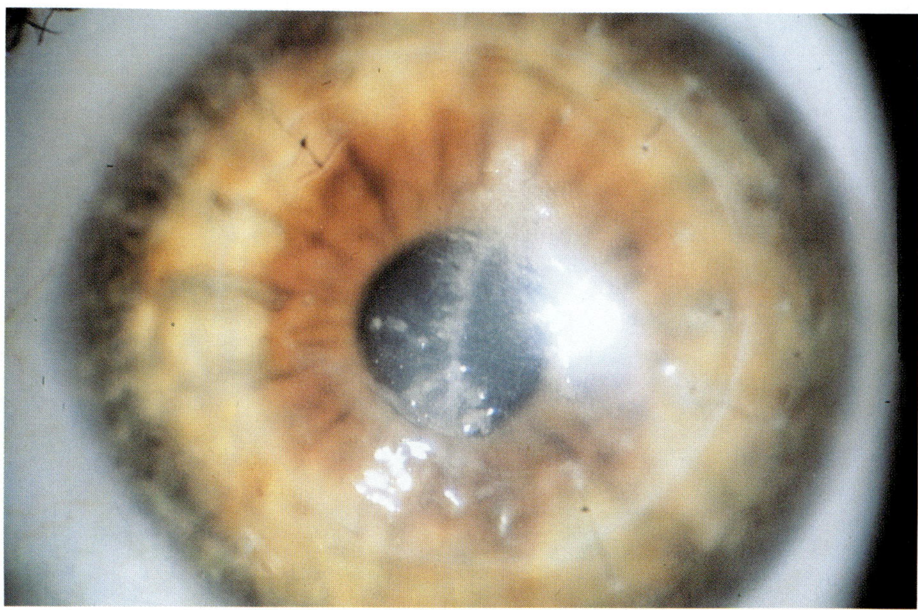

A

Figure 5–6. Case 19. **(A)** A 41-year-old woman with recurrent lattice dystrophy in a corneal graft. Note the irregular corneal surface and thick ropy lattice deposits beneath the epithelium and in the superficial corneal stroma. Visual acuity is 20/80. *(Continued on following page)*

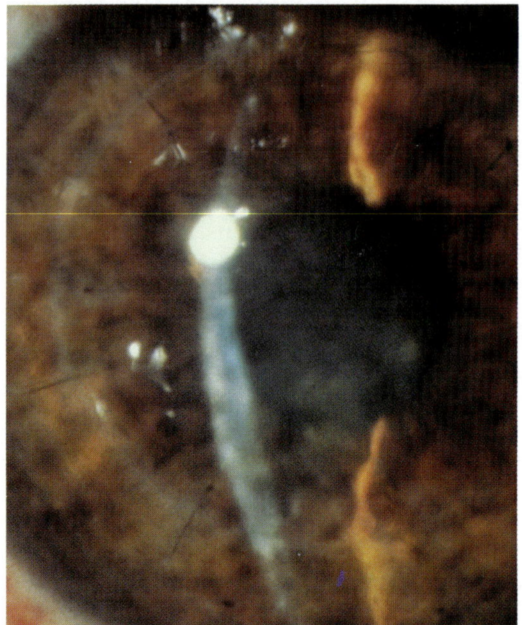

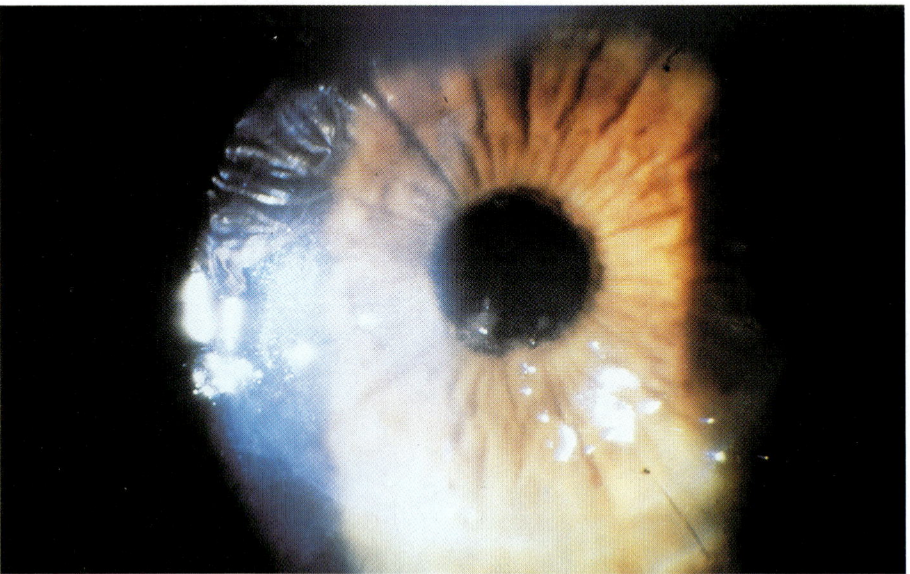

Figure 5–6 (B).   Graft rejection episode 2 weeks following excimer laser PTK. Inferiorly, note thickened slit beam denoting graft edema. An endothelial rejection line is faintly visible. Visual acuity is 20/200. (Reprinted with permission from Hersh et al.[19]) **(C)** Following treatment with corticosteroids, the graft has cleared without adverse sequelae. The cornea has a smooth surface and improved clarity with return of visual acuity to 20/25 following PTK.

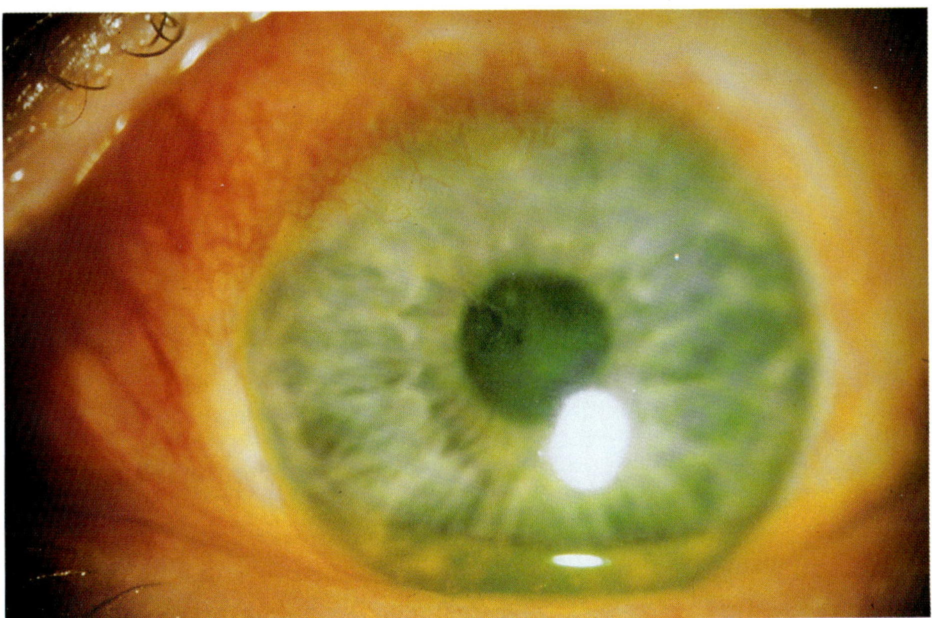

Figure 5–7.   Case 20. A 60-year-old man with anterior stromal scarring secondary to a 20 year history of herpes simplex keratitis. Corrected spectacle visual acuity was 20/400. PTK was performed after a preoperative quiescent period of 1 year. Postoperative treatment included trifluridine, combined tobramycin and dexamethasone, and pressure patching. After re-epithelialization, treatment with trifluridine and prednisolone acetate was maintained. Three months after treatment, there was a recurrence of herpes simplex dendritic keratitis. This was treated by increasing antiviral medications and tapering corticosteroid eyedrops with a resolution of the dendritic keratitis in several weeks. Visual acuity improved to 20/70. (Photo courtesy of Michael P. Vrabec, M.D. Reproduced with permission from Vrabec et al.[18])

Herpes keratitis is thus a relative contraindication for PTK. PTK should not be performed on eyes with active herpes simplex virus. If subsequently performed, a quiescent period of 6–12 months is preferred preoperatively. In addition, perioperative treatment with topical antiviral agents (e.g., trifluridine), as well as oral acyclovir, may act as prophylaxis against recurrent herpetic infection.

Recurrence of Disease

Patients with corneal dytrophies or degenerations undergoing PTK may suffer recurrences following the procedure. Disorders such as lattice dystrophy, epithelial basement membrane dystrophy, Salzmann's nodular degeneration, and others may recur at variable intervals following the procedure. It is important to advise the patient of this possibility. PTK or manual superficial keratectomy, while clearing and smoothing the cornea, does not correct the underlying disorder of the epithelium or keratocytes. Thus, with time, the disease process may again present itself. In such cases, PTK (or superficial keratectomy) can be repeated.

CASE 21

A 24-year-old woman with Reis-Buckler's corneal dystrophy underwent manual superficial keratectomy OU in 1990 with improvement of best-corrected visual acuity from 20/80 to 20/40 (Fig. 5–8). When seen again in 1993, visual acuity had again decreased to 20/100 OD and 20/80 OS secondary to recurrence of the dystrophy. PTK was performed with improvement in best-corrected visual acuity to 20/30. Two years later, the dystrophy again recurred, with a decrease in best-corrected visual acuity to 20/80. Preoperative pachymetry demonstrated a corneal thickness of 580 μm. PTK was repeated with improvement in visual acuity to 20/40. Corneal thickness was decreased to 488 μm.

This case demonstrates the ability of PTK to re-treat recurrent disease. Retreatment, however, may be limited by the residual corneal thickness. Corneas thinner than 400 μm should be treated with caution for fear of inducing ectasia or damage to the corneal endothelium with very deep laser ablations. In such cases, manual keratectomy or keratoplasty may be an alternative.

Subsequent Penetrating Keratoplasty

Although one of the important goals of PTK is to obviate the need for penetrating keratoplasty, keratoplasty may still be necessary in some cases. There is no evidence to date that corneas following PTK are technically more difficult on which to perform surgery nor does there seem to be any decrease in success of penetrating keratoplasty following the excimer laser procedure.[2] In one study of 232 eyes,[8] 3 eyes subsequently underwent penetrating keratoplasty.

Refractive and Topography Changes

This group of complications is discussed in Chapter 6.

Conclusions

The complications associated with PTK comprise those resulting from corneal surgery in general, in addition to topography and refractive considerations. Patients should be carefully followed for persistent epithelial defects, and associated complications should be promptly treated.

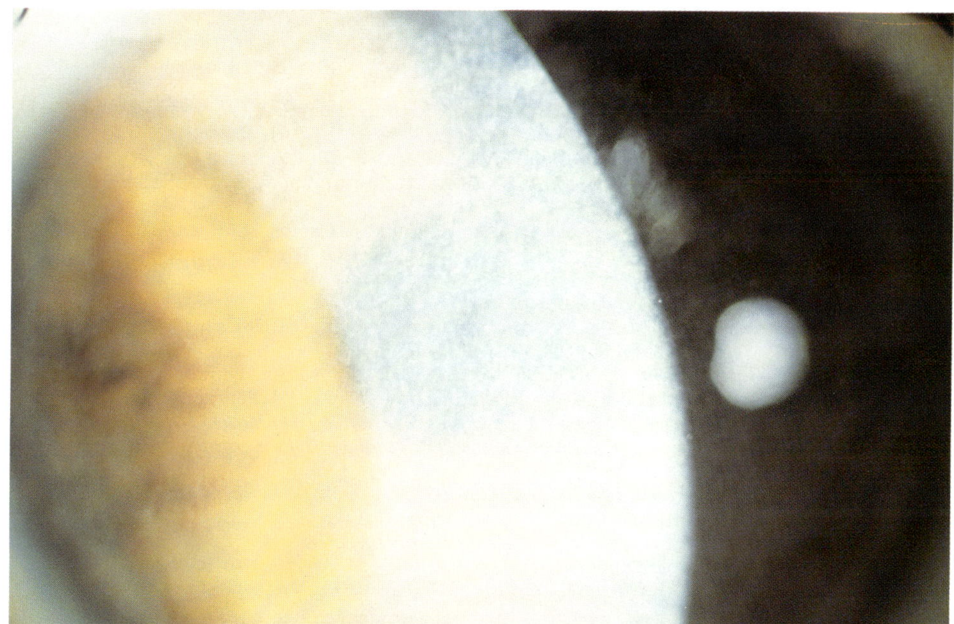

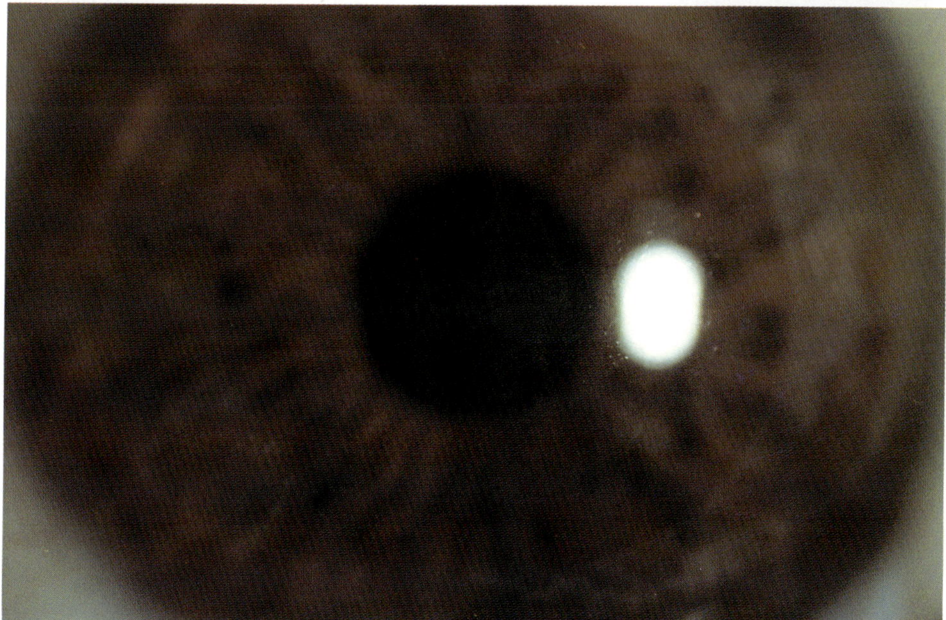

Figure 5–8.   Case 21. Three years following superficial keratectomy, Reis-Buckler's corneal dystrophy had recurred, and spectacle corrected visual acuity had decreased to 20/100. Following PTK, best-corrected visual acuity improved to 20/30. **(A)** Two years later, the dystrophy has again recurred, with a decrease in spectacle corrected visual acuity to 20/80. **(B)** Repeat PTK is rewarded by improvement in visual acuity to 20/40.

References

1. Kenyon KR, Tseng SCG. Limbal autograft transplantation for ocular surface disorders. Ophthalmology 1989;96:709–723.
2. Hersh PS, Burnstein Y, Carr J, Etwaru G, Mayers M. Phototherapeutic keratectomy: surgical strategies and clinical outcomes. Ophthalmology 1996;103:1210–1222.
3. Badr IA, Al-Rajhi A, Wagoner MD, Dunham T, Teichmann KD, Cameron JA, and the KKESH Excimer Laser Study Group. Phototherapeutic keratectomy for climatic droplet keratopathy. J Refract Surg 1996;12:114–122.
4. Gangadhar D, Kenyon KR, Wagoner MD. Superficial keratectomy. In W Tasman, EA Jaeger (eds): Duane's Clinical Ophthalmology. Vol. 6. Philadelphia: JB Lippincott, 1994.
5. Al-Rajhi A, Wagoner MD, Badr IA, Al-Saif A, Mahmood M. Bacterial keratitis following phototherapeutic keratectomy. J Refract Surg 1996;12:123–127.
6. Fulton JC, Cohen EJ, Rapuano CJ. Bacterial ulcer 3 days after excimer laser phototherapeutic keratectomy. Arch Ophthalmol 1996;114:626–627.
7. Fagerholm P, Fitzsimmons TD, Orndahl M, Ohman L, Tengroth B. Phototherapeutic keratectomy: long term results in 166 eyes. J Refract Corneal Surg 1993;9(suppl):s76–81.
8. Maloney RK, Thompson V, Ghiselli G, Durrie D, Waring GO, O'Connell M. A prospective multicenter trial of excimer laser phototherapeutic keratectomy for corneal vision loss. Am J Ophthalmol 1996;122:149–160.
9. Teichmann KD, Cameron J, Huaman A, Rahi AHS, Badr I. Wellely-type immune ring following phototherapeutic keratectomy. J Cataract Refract Surg 1996;22:142–146.
10. Ormerod DL, Dahan E, Hagele JE, Guzek JP. Serious occurrences in the natural history of advanced climatic droplet keratopathy. Ophthalmology 1994;101:448–453.
11. Al-Hazzaa S, Tabbara KF. Bacterial keratitis after penetrating keratoplasty. Ophthalmology 1986;95:1504–1508.
12. Tavakkoli H, Sugar J. Microbial keratitis following penetrating keratoplasty. Ophthalmic Surg 1994;25:356–360.
13. Varley GA, Meisler DM. Complications of penetrating keratoplasty: graft infections. J Refract Corneal Surg 1991;7:62–66.
14. Fong LP, Ormerod LD, Kenyon KR, Foster CS. Microbial keratitis complicating penetrating keratoplasty. Ophthalmology 1988;95:1269–1275.
15. Gorovoy MS, Stern GA, Hood CI, Allen C. Intrastromal noninflammatory colonization of a corneal graft. Arch Ophthalmol 1983;101:1749–1752.
16. Epstein RJ, Robin JB. Corneal graft rejection episode after excimer laser phototherapeutic keratectomy [letter]. Arch Ophthalmol 1994;112:157.
17. Vrabec MP, Anderson JA, Rock ME et al. Electron microscopic findings in a cornea with recurrence of herpes simplex keratitis after excimer laser phototherapeutic keratectomy. CLAO J 1994;20:41–44.
18. Vrabec MP, Durrie DS, Chase DS. Recurrence of herpes simplex after excimer laser keratectomy. Am J Ophthalmol 1992;114:96–97.
19. Hersh PS, Jordan AJ, Mayers M. Corneal graft resection episode after excimer laser phototherapeutic keratectomy. Arch Ophthamol 1993;111:735–736.

♦ 6 ♦

Refractive and Topographic Complications and Considerations

In addition to the complications discussed in Chapter 5, changes in corneal curvature may lead to refractive shifts after PTK. Such effects may be predicted by the type of corneal disorder treated and the surgical strategy employed. The anticipated refractive changes, therefore, should be considered during the case selection process.

Changes in Corneal Topography

PTK is performed in many cases to improve surface irregularity. It may also be used in an attempt to correct irregular astigmatism per se (see Chapter 3).[1] Thus, topography would be expected to improve in many cases. Indeed, in one study of 28 eyes,[2] corneal topography was graded as improved in 17 eyes (61%), remained unchanged in 10 (36%), and worsened in 1 (4%). The last patient had been treated for a superficial stromal scar and required a rigid contact lens to attain best-corrected visual acuity postoperatively (Fig. 6–1).

In another study of 83 eyes examined 6 months after PRK,[3] corneal surface smoothness was rated on a scale of 0 to 3 (0 = most regular, 3 = most irregular). The average preoperative surface irregularity was 1.8. Surface smoothness improved in 59 eyes (71%), remained the same in 22 eyes (27%), and worsened in 2 eyes (2%).

Case 22

HISTORY AND PREOPERATIVE EVALUATION

An 80-year-old man with Salzmann's nodular degeneration complained of monocular diplopia and photophobia (Fig. 6–2). On examination, the monocular diplopia disappeared when the nodules were covered by the edge of a card. Visual acuity was 20/40. On slit-lamp examination, two nodules were present, measuring approximately 2.0 and 1.5 mm, respectively. Videokeratoscopy demonstrated focal irregularity superiorly at rings 1–4 overlying the corneal nodules and steepening over the nodules.

SURGICAL THERAPY AND OUTCOME

The epithelium was removed with dry cellulose sponges over the nodules themselves, but left in place over the areas of clear cornea. The laser beam diameter was set for 2.0 mm, and laser was applied until the level of the nodule was lowered to the normal corneal surface. Following focal PTK, the monocular diplopia and photophobia resolved. The videokeratoscope image was more regular, and the corresponding topographic map showed marked improvement in the corneal steepening with a decrease in irregular astigmatism. Postoperative visual acuity was 20/25.

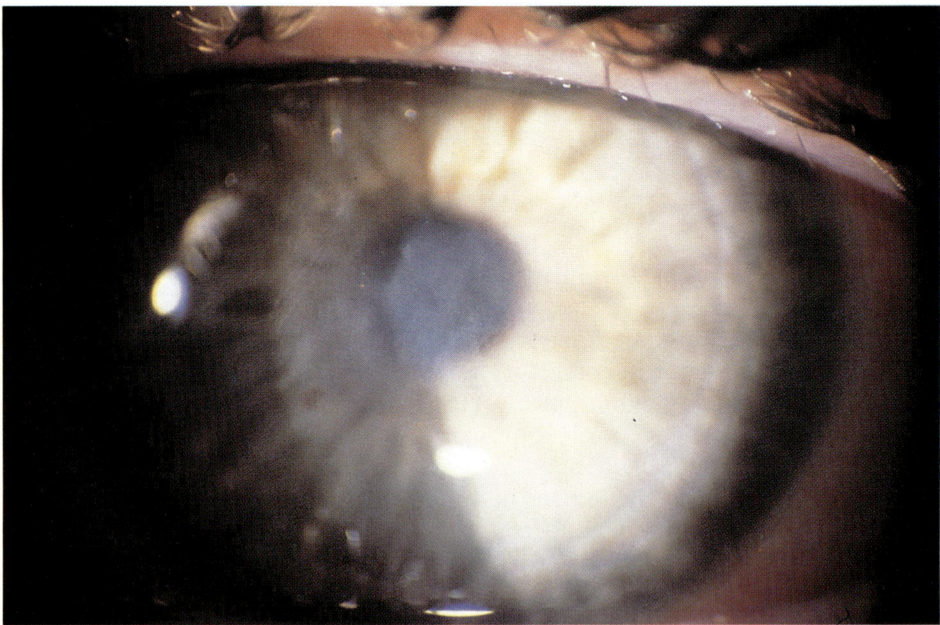

A

Figure 6–1.   Case 25. **(A)** A 32-year-old woman with inactive scar following herpes simplex keratitis. Visual acuity is 20/60. *(Continued on following page)*

B

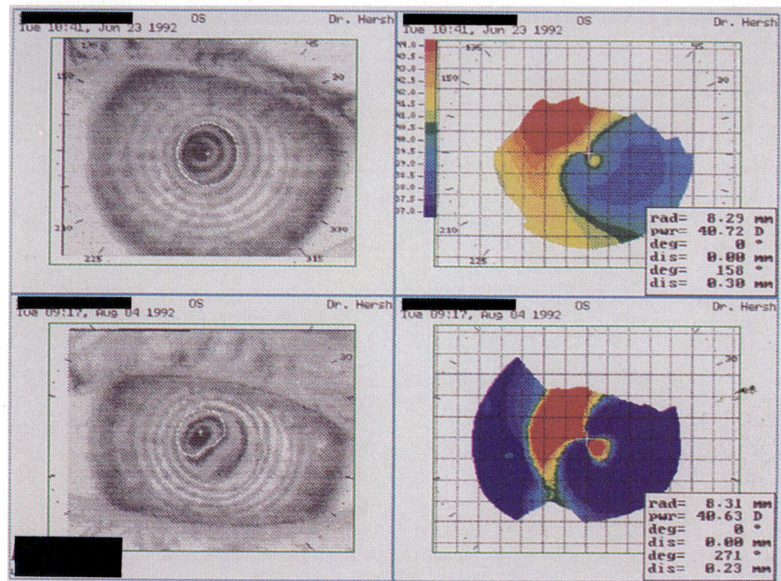

C

Figure 6–1 (B).   Immediately following PTK, the cornea is clear but with surface irregularity. **(C, top left and right)** Preoperative videokeratoscope image and corresponding topographic map. **(C, bottom left and right)** One month following treatment, the corneal surface overlying the ablated area shows increased irregularity with induction of irregular astigmatism. Best-corrected spectacle visual acuity has decreased to 20/100 but improves to 20/50 with a rigid gas-permeable contact lens.

Case 23

HISTORY AND PREOPERATIVE EVALUATION

A 41-year-old man suffered eye trauma many years earlier (Fig. 6–3). On examination, a plaquelike, fibrous corneal scar was seen to extend from the nasal periphery over the visual axis. Visual acuity was 20/100.

SURGICAL THERAPY AND OUTCOME

Given the plaquelike nature of the scar, a combined focal manual keratectomy and PTK was performed. After initial manual keratectomy, only 96 laser pulses at 4.0 mm and 40 pulses at 3.0 mm were necessary to achieve desired corneal smoothing and clearing. After surgery, the cornea appeared clearer, and visual acuity had improved to 20/25. Videokeratography showed a marked improvement in surface smoothness.

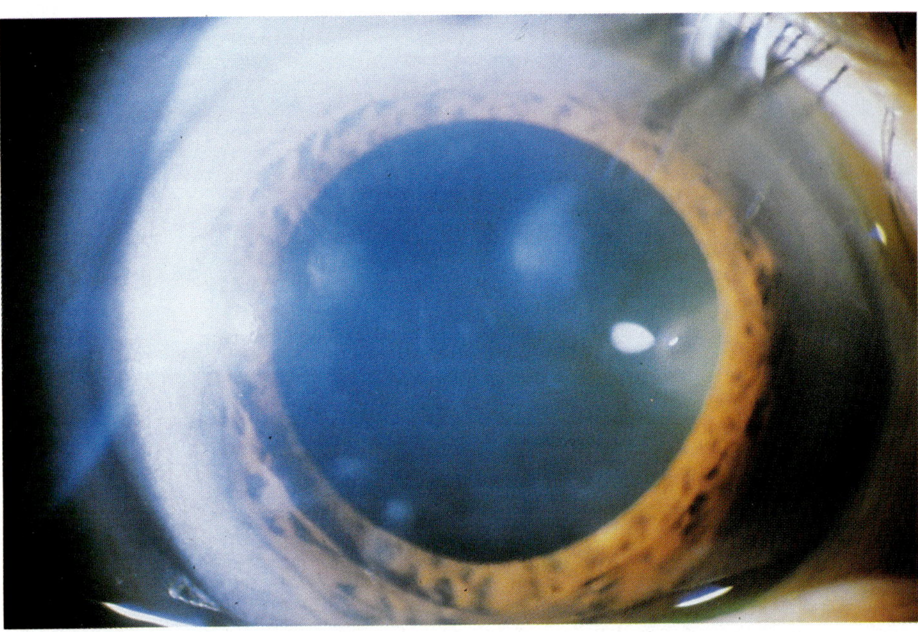

A

Figure 6–2.   Case 22. **(A)** An 80-year-old man with Salzmann's nodular degeneration complained of monocular diplopia and photophobia. Visual acuity is 20/40. **(B)** Following focal excimer laser smoothing of the superior nodules, the monocular diplopia and photophobia have resolved. Visual acuity is 20/25. **(C, top left)** Videokeratoscope image before PTK shows focal irregularity superiorly at rings 1–4 overlying corneal nodule. **(C, top right)** Corresponding topographic map demonstrating corneal steepening over the nodule. **(C, bottom left)** Following focal PTK, the videokeratoscope image is more regular. **(C, bottom right)** Corresponding topographic map shows marked improvement in the corneal steepening with decrease in irregular astigmatism. *(Continued on following page)*

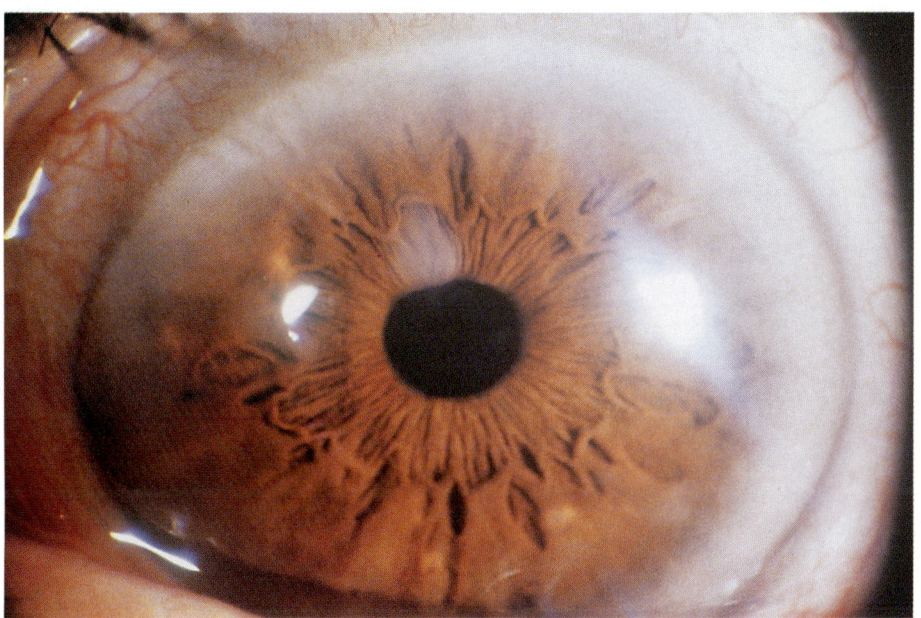

Figure 6–2 (B)

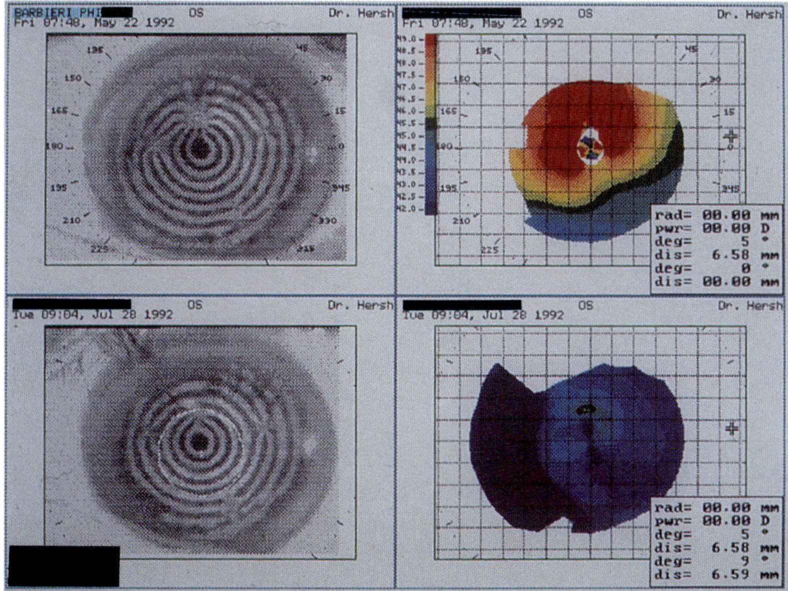

Figure 6–2 (C)

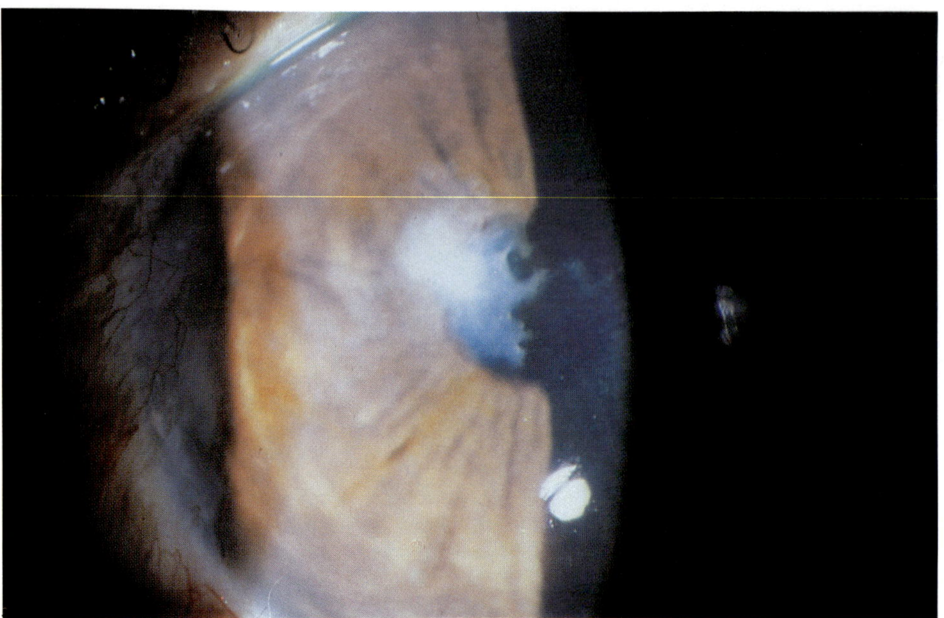

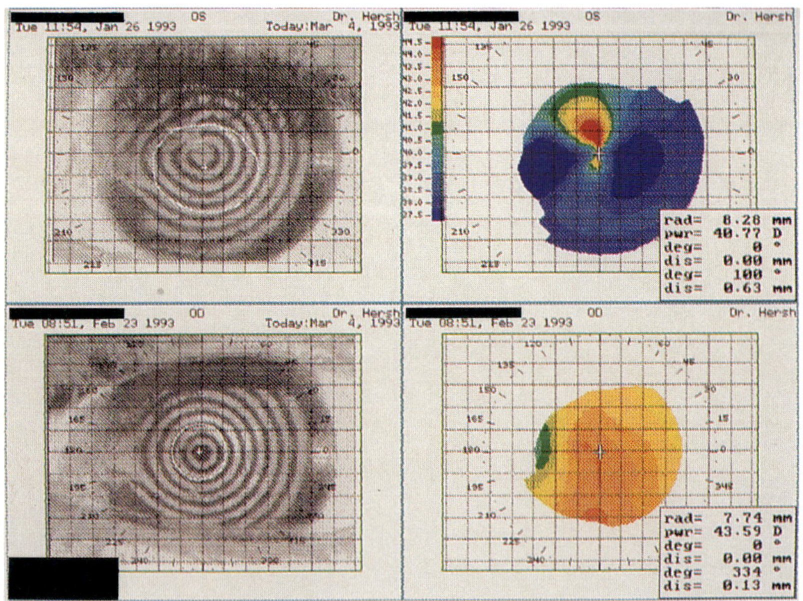

Figure 6–3.   Case 23. **(A)** A 41-year-old man suffered eye trauma many years earlier. On examination, a plaquelike, fibrous corneal scar was seen to extend from the nasal periphery over the visual axis. Visual acuity was 20/100. **(B)** Videokeratography before **(top)** and after **(bottom)** surgery shows a marked improvement in surface smoothness.

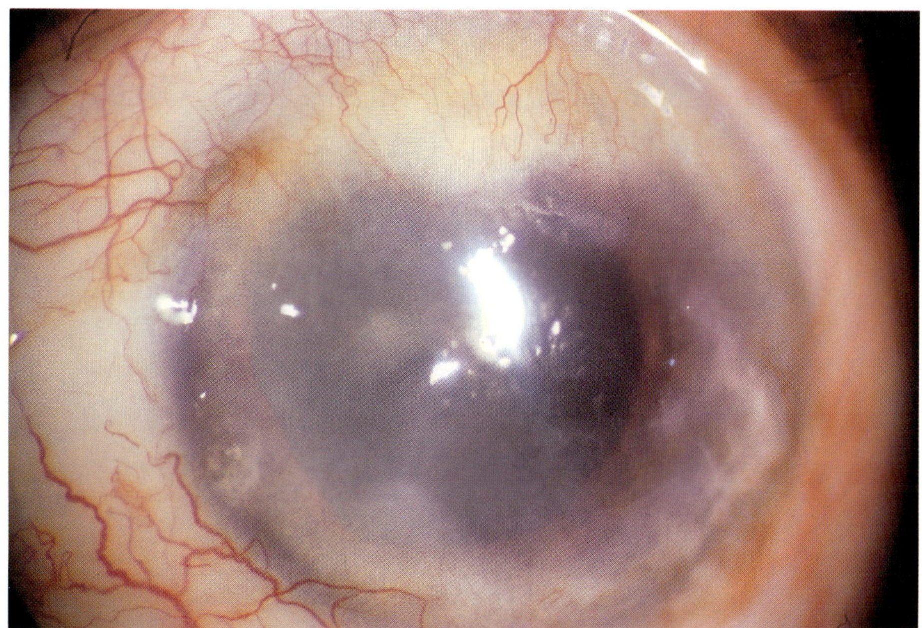

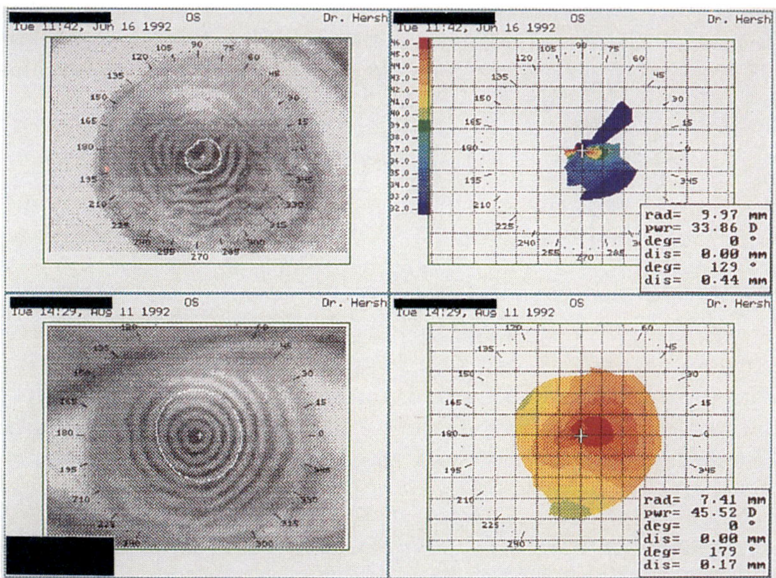

Figure 6–4.   Case 24. **(A)** Preoperative appearance of a 70-year-old woman showing corneal degenerative changes and a markedly irregular surface. Visual acuity is 20/400. **(B)** Following general large area PTK, the cornea cleared with some remaining haze, the surface smoothed, and visual acuity increased to 20/50. Videokeratography before **(top)** and after **(bottom)** PTK shows improved corneal surface smoothness.

Case 24

HISTORY AND PREOPERATIVE EVALUATION

A 70-year-old woman with visual acuity of 20/400 had a long-standing peripheral and central corneal degeneration with a markedly irregular corneal surface (Fig. 6–4).

SURGICAL THERAPY AND OUTCOME

A general large area PTK using 500 laser pulses at 5.0 mm and 123 pulses at 3.5 mm was performed. Following surgery, the cornea had cleared with some remaining haze, the surface had smoothed, and visual acuity increased to 20/50. Videokeratography demonstrated a markedly improved corneal surface smoothness.

Case 25

HISTORY AND PREOPERATIVE EVALUATION

A 32-year-old woman with inactive scar following herpes simplex keratitis was seen with a best-corrected visual acuity of 20/60 (Fig. 6–1). Uncorrected visual acuity was 20/200. On slit-lamp examination, there was a central corneal scar measuring approximately 5 mm. The depth of the scar was approximately 15% of the corneal thickness. The corneal epithelial surface appeared smooth. Corneal thickness as measured by ultrasonic pachometry was 498 µm. Computer-assisted videokeratography showed moderate irregularity with flattening over the scar.

ALGORITHMIC ANALYSIS

Horizontal assessment. The pathology is in the central optical zone (green color code), allowing consideration of possible PTK, pending further analysis of other parameters.

Pattern of pathology. In this case, there is diffuse anterior stromal pathology in the center of the cornea, extending into the stromal substance itself. Based on the location and depth of the scar, the smoothness of the epithelium, and the confirmatory computerized corneal topography of moderate irregular astigmatism, the approach selected was transepithelial PTK to remove the scar.

SURGICAL THERAPY AND OUTCOME

PTK was performed employing a transepithelial technique. A polishing technique was chosen with adjunctive use of methylcellulose 1% as a masking solution. A 5.0 mm beam diameter was used for a total of 378 pulses followed by 149 pulses at 3.0 mm to smooth the junction of the treated and nontreated cornea. Immediately following PTK, the cornea was clear with good removal of the scar. Postoperative epithelial healing was without complication. However, uncorrected visual acuity remained 20/200, and spectacle-corrected visual acuity was 20/100, decreasing from the preoperative value. Visual acuity with a rigid contact lens was 20/50. On videokeratography, the cornea surface overlying the ablated area showed increased irregularity with induction of irregular astigmatism and further corneal flattening.

DISCUSSION

This case exemplifies adverse topography changes that can occur with a corneal scar located within the stromal substance itself. In retrospect, although a polishing technique was used, too much tissue was removed from the scarred area, inducing irregular astigmatism with a decrease in spectacle corrected visual acuity.

Refractive Shifts

Of great importance in case selection and surgical technique is the recognition of changes in refraction that may result from the PTK procedure. Although PTK is generally performed with a laser beam of constant diameter without a refractive correction programmed into the laser's computer, corneal shape changes frequently lead to refractive shifts following the procedure. In particular, significant corneal flattening should be anticipated with some types of PTK treatment. In one study,[2] for instance, treated eyes showed a mean spherical equivalent refractive change of +1.4 diopters with a range of −5.25 to +7.25 diopters. A hyperopic shift of >1.0 diopters was observed in 10 eyes (40%) with a mean change in these patients of +4.8 diopters. A myopic shift of >1.0 diopters was noted in 3 eyes (12%) with a mean change of −4.76 diopters. Table 6–1 shows the refractive shifts stratified to treatment strategy in that study. Patients receiving general large area PTK, combined superficial keratectomy and PTK, and superficial scar removal showed mean hyperopic shifts of >2 diopters. Those with focal smoothing and treatment for epithelial basement membrane dystrophy showed only mild refractive changes. Of those patients with refractive shifts, a shift toward emmetropia was observed in 15 eyes, while a shift away from emmetropia was noted in 10 eyes.

In another multicenter study of 103 eyes using the Summit excimer laser,[3] there was a mean hyperopic shift of +0.87 diopters. In this study, the maximal hyperopic change was +8.5 diopters, and the maximal myopic change was −5.5 diopters. Forty percent of eyes had a hyperopic change of 1.0 diopters or more and 21% had a myopic change of 1.0 diopters or more. The investigators found that the mean spherical equivalent refraction stabilized 3 months following surgery. However, they noted some eyes with varying refraction afterward, with 22 (24%) of 92 eyes changing by 1.0 diopter or more between postoperative months 6 and 12.

In 18 eyes treated using the VisX laser,[4] a hyperopic shift was observed in 10 eyes (56%). These eyes were treated by performing a disk-shaped ablation

Table 6–1. Refractive Shift Following PTK

TECHNIQUE	NO. OF EYES	MEAN REFRACTIVE CHANGE	MEAN NO. OF LASER PULSES	MEAN CHANGE IN CORNEAL THICKNESS (MICRONS)	WITHIN ±1.0 DIOPTER OF PREOPERATIVE REFRACTION	NO. OF EYES	
						HYPEROPIC (>1.00 D)	*MYOPIC (>1.00 D)*
General large area PTK	7	+2.9 D	643	46	2	4	1
PTK with superficial keratectomy	2	+4.1 D	498	110	1	1	0
Focal smoothing	6	−0.5 D	296	36	4	1	1
Scar removal	5	+2.7 D	524	69	1	4	0
EBMD/RES*	5	+0.7 D	36	1	4	0	1
Total	25	+1.4 D	418	31	12	10 (40%)	3 (12%)

*Epithelial basement membrane dystrophy/recurrent erosion syndrome.
(Reproduced with permission from Hersh et al.[2] Courtesy of Ophthalmology.)

of uniform depth depending on the preoperative thickness of the corneal pathology as measured by optical pachymetry. Neither a polishing nor a peripheral smoothing technique (see Chapter 3) was used. The mean refractive shift was +7.05 diopters at 1 month and +6.45 diopters at 3 months postoperatively. Refractive shifts in this study could not be correlated with disease process.

In a study of 33 eyes using the Taunton Technologies excimer laser, a hyperopic shift was found in approximately 50% of patients.[5]

Case 26

HISTORY AND PREOPERATIVE EVALUATION

A 31-year-old woman with Reis-Buckler's dystrophy had a best-corrected vision of 20/200 with a refraction of −6.50 dioptors and uncorrected visual acuity of counts fingers (Fig. 6–5).

SURGICAL THERAPY AND OUTCOME

A large area general PTK technique was used. Treatment comprised 1,065 pulses with use of methylcellulose 1% as a masking compound. Postopera-

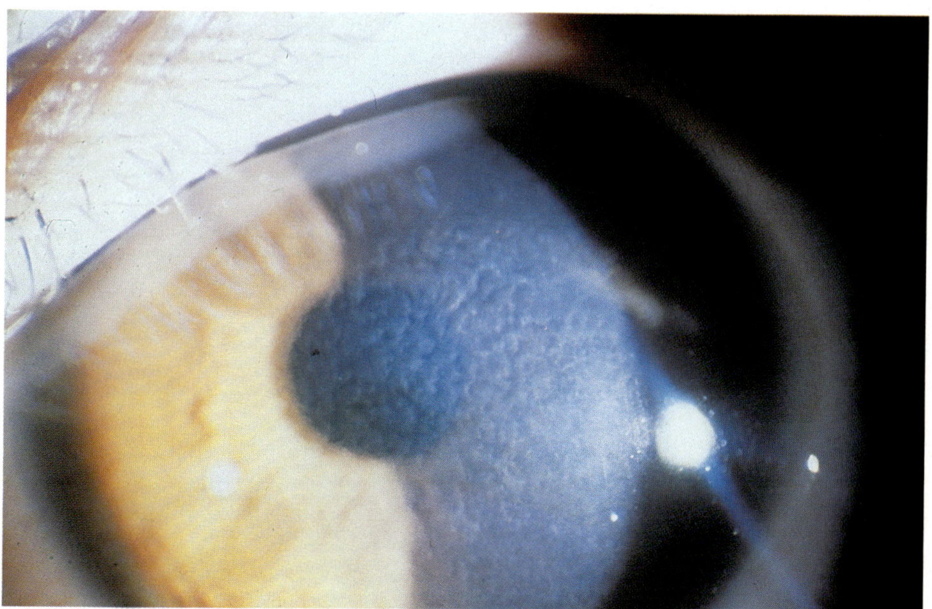

Figure 6–5.   Case 26. **(A)** Preoperative appearance of a 31-year-old woman with Reis-Buckler's dystrophy and best-corrected vision of 20/200 with a refraction of −6.50. (*Continued on following page*)

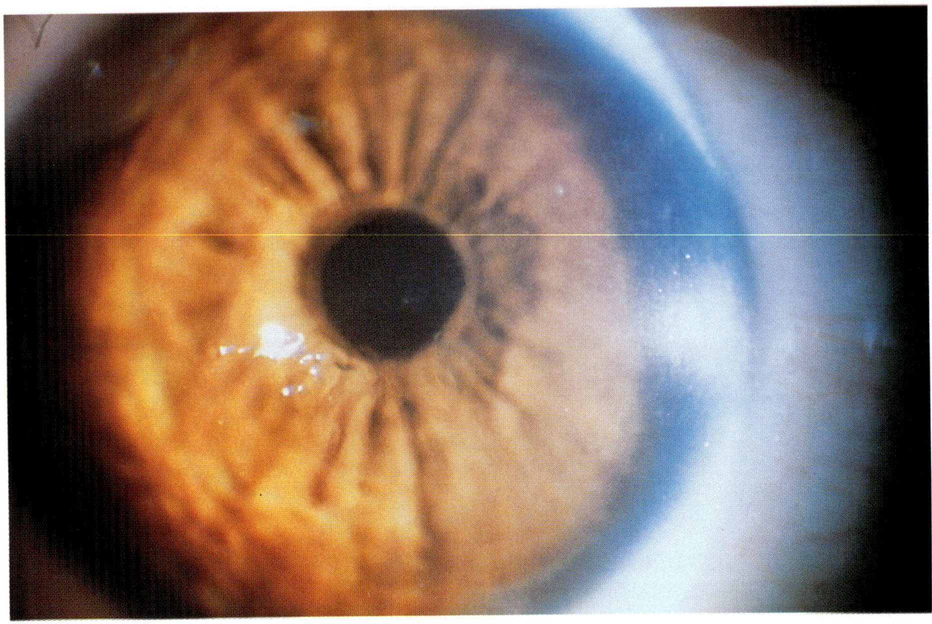

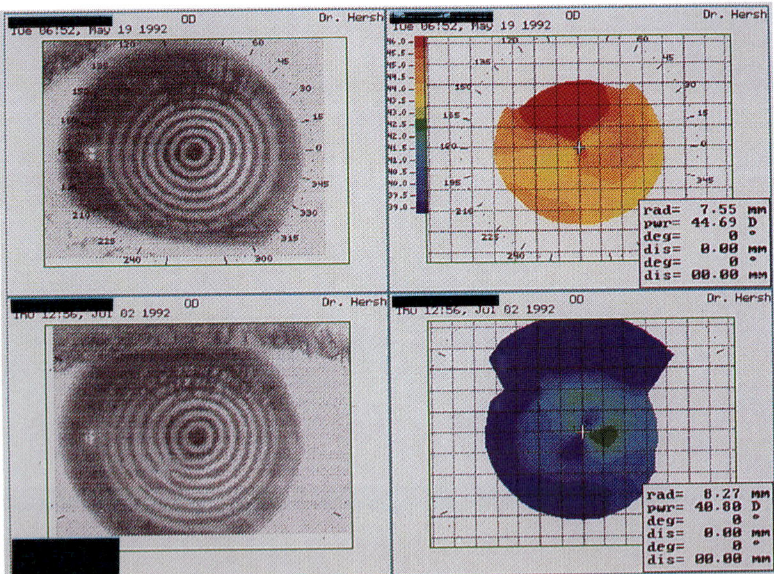

Figure 6–5 (B). Postoperatively, the cornea is clear with restoration of best-corrected spectacle vision to 20/30. The refraction is −2.50, showing a 4 diopter hyperopic shift. **(C)** Videokeratography before **(top)** and after **(bottom)** PTK showing marked flattening of the cornea.

tively, the cornea was much clearer with restoration of best-corrrected spectacle vision to 20/30. However, the refraction was −2.50, showing a 4 diopter hyperopic shift.

DISCUSSION

This patient demonstrates a substantial hyperopic shift that, in her case of significant preoperative myopia, was not undesirable. Other family members were evaluated. The patient's father, for instance, showed similar Reis-Buckler's dystrophy with a significant deficit in vision. However, his refractive error preoperatively was +5.0 diopters. Therefore, PTK was deferred for fear of substantial and intolerable postoperative hyperopia.

Mechanism of Refractive Shifts

When performing PTK, the laser beam is of fixed diameter. Since the energy profile of the laser beam is optimally homogenous over its face, the ablation rate would theoretically be similar over the treated area of the cornea. Thus, with a direct ablation without polishing, the surface optical profile would be expected to be preserved without a change in corneal power or topography, and the refraction similarly would be expected to be unchanged. Studies and practice indicate that this is not the case, however. Hyperopic shifting is a frequent concomitant of the PTK procedure. There are several hypotheses attempting to explain the refractive shifts seen (Fig. 6–6).

First, the induced corneal flattening may be caused by an unequal postoperative epithelial thickness with the creation of an epithelial lens power different from the curvature of the underlying treated stroma.[6,7] In the case of corneal flattening, for instance, epithelial hyperplasia at the periphery of the treated area could be implicated as a cause for this hyperopic shifting.

Second, the theoretically perfect excimer laser beam would have a consistent radiant energy density in all dimensions.[8] In this case, given a homogeneous cornea without ablation resistent areas and without the introduction of masking compounds such as methycellulose,[9] the corneal curvature would be expected to be preserved without a resulting refractive change. However, the beam in practice may exhibit a somewhat attenuated fluence at its peripheral aspect. Thus the peripheral ablation rate may be slightly less militating toward corneal flattening.

Third, of theoretical effect, though of questionable clinical impact, is the changing angle of incidence of the beam across the central corneal dome. This would result in a lower fluence peripherally with a decrease in effective tissue ablation and consequent corneal flattening.[10]

Finally, other investigators[11] suggest that removal of central portions of the corneal stromal lamellae may lead to centrifugal differential contraction of the remaining lamellae with consequent central flattening. The same authors

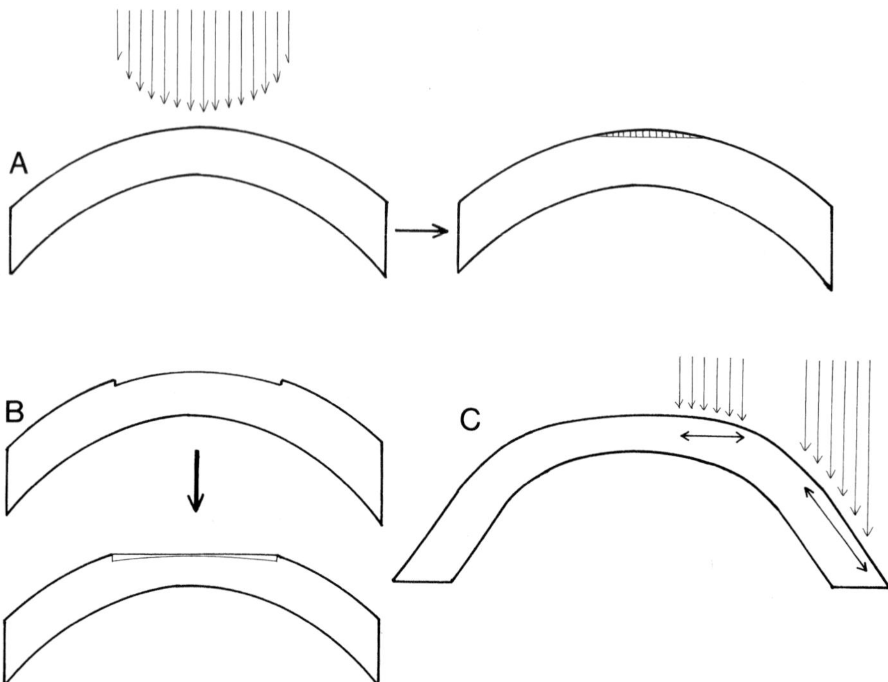

Figure 6–6. Possible factors contributing to refractive shifts with PTK. **(A)** Attenuation of laser fluence toward the periphery of the beam resulting in relatively less tissue removal peripherally than centrally, with focal corneal flattening in the area of treatment. Note that this flattening is exaggerated. **(B)** Relative epithelial hyperplasia at the peripheral aspect of the treatment zone leading to corneal surface flattening, although the stromal curvature remains unchanged. **(C)** The changing angle of incidence of the beam across the corneal dome results in a lower fluence peripherally, decreasing the effective tissue ablation peripherally and leading to flattening.

also speculate that the laser effluent plume may differentially block the periphery of the incoming beam, thus leading to less peripheral ablation. Moreover, they suggest that it is unlikely that the degree of flattening seen is a consequence solely of inhomogeneities in the laser beam.

Aside from these laser-related causes, other investigators[12] speculate that some of the induced refractive change in Reis-Buckler's dystrophy, for instance, may simply result from the excision of the abnormal subepithelial tissue whether by a laser or manual superficial keratectomy technique.

The location of the corneal pathology and, thus, the laser treatment may also be important in determining consequent refractive changes. Flattening may occur with treatment of the central cornea. Steepening, in contrast, may occur when more tissue is ablated peripherally than centrally. Although this may flatten the focal areas of cornea treated due the the mechanisms discussed above,[1] the overall macroscopic optical contour of the cornea may steepen if peripheral tissue is removed (Fig. 6–7).

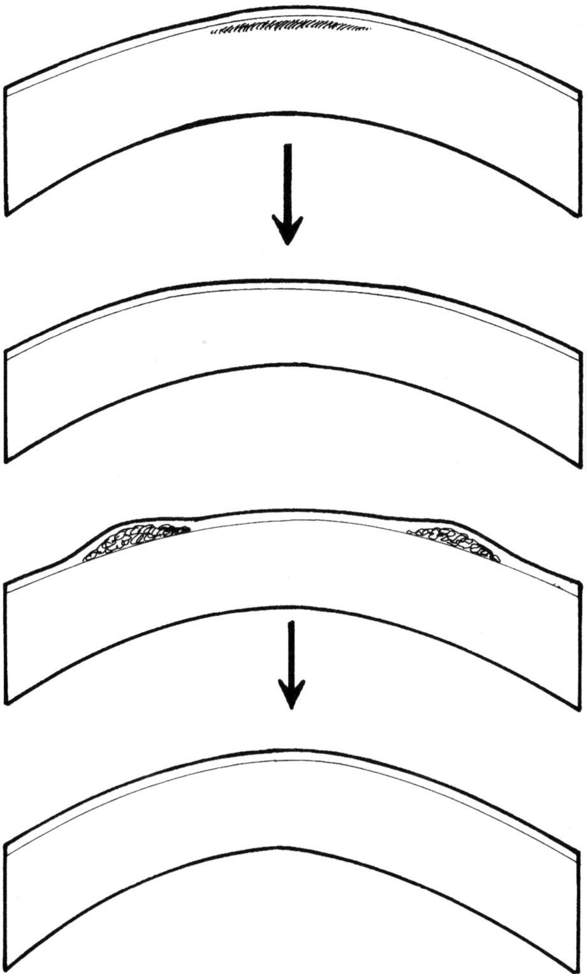

Figure 6–7.   Treatment of central cornea leading to flattening of the corneal surface. (Top) Treatment of the peripheral cornea leading to steepening of the overall corneal contour. (Bottom)

Minimizing Refractive Shifts and Topographic Changes

Refractive changes should always be anticipated when selecting patients for PTK.[8] Shifts away from emmetropia may be undesirable, leaving the patient unacceptably anisometropic or hyperopic. In general, some degree of induced flattening should be anticipated for most PTK procedures performed on the central cornea, while either central flattening or steepening may occur with more peripheral treatments, such as smoothing of scars and irregularities following pterygium surgery.

To avoid these complications, deep stromal scars with the removal of a large amount of corneal stromal tissue should be avoided. Protruding surface excrescenses such as Salzmann's nodules are best. Treatment of the former will often result in perturbation of the corneal topography, while ablation of the latter will result in smoothing and regularization of the surface topography with reattainment of the normal corneal curvature.

During treatment, refractive shifts likely may be minimized by blending the treatment zone using the techniques described in Chapter 3 and, importantly, by limiting the actual amount of tissue ablated. In addition, performing an annular peripheral treatment with a small beam diameter at the conclusion of the PTK may smooth the junction of the treated and untreated cornea and, thus, mitigate against hyperopic shifts (see Chapter 3).

Technique of "Hyperopic" PTK

As discussed in Chapter 3, there is a surgical strategy which attempts to directly circumvent hyperopic shifts and may even result in slight myopic shifting. In this technique, a wide beam diameter (usually $\geq$6.0 mm) is used to directly ablate the cornea without movement of the patient's head. The treatment is centered on the pupil rather than the scar itself to avoid postoperative optical zone edge effects. The number of pulses may be estimated by the depth of the corneal scar as measured by optical pachymetry (number of pulses = depth of scar in microns $\times$ 4), but should be minimized for safety. The epithelium may be removed manually or with the laser.

Upon satisfactory removal of the scar (as monitored by slit lamp examination), the center of the cornea over the pupil is physically masked. Masking may be accomplished by using a small trephine (4.0 to 5.0 mm) to cut a disc from a sterile disposable soft contact lens. The contact lens disc is then placed, centered over the pupil. A disc of sterile filter paper or a drop of methylcellulose 2.5% may similarly accomplish the masking of the central cornea. However, the contact lens mask is easy to fashion, is sterile, and remains in position best during the subsequent laser treatment.

After application of the corneal mask, and without changing the laser beam diameter, additional treatment (approximately 50 to 100 pulses) is applied. Since the central laser beam is blocked by the mask on the cornea, a peripheral "hyperopic" annulus of tissue removal measuring 1.0 to 1.5 mm in diameter is created. When the cornea subsequently re-epithelializes, hyperopic shifting thus should be minimized since the peripheral annulus will tend to steepen the overall corneal contour (Fig. 3–26, Fig. 6–8, Case 12, Case 27, Case 28).

In the near future, excimer lasers that are able to perform hyperopic corrections directly may provide a refined methodology of this technique, and be used on a routine basis as part of the PTK procedure to avoid induced corneal flattening.

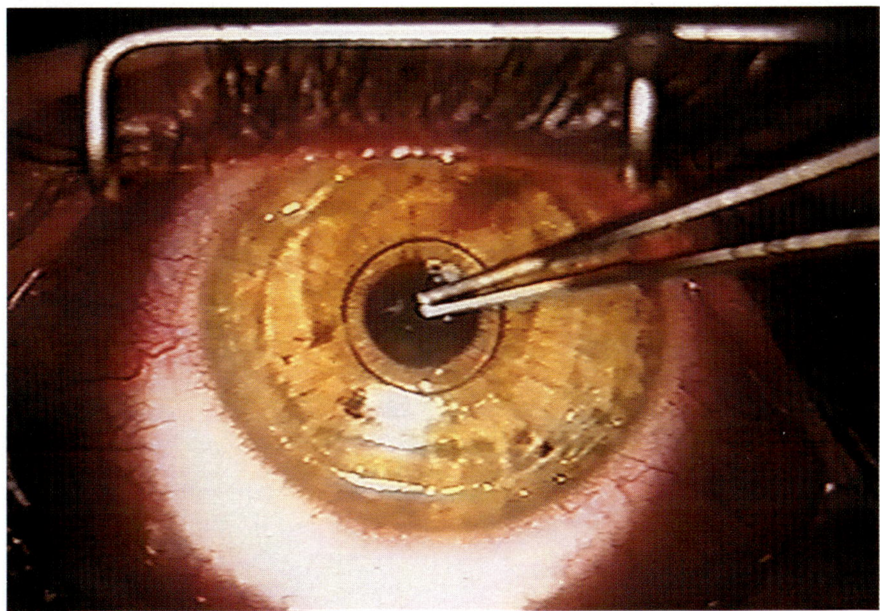

A

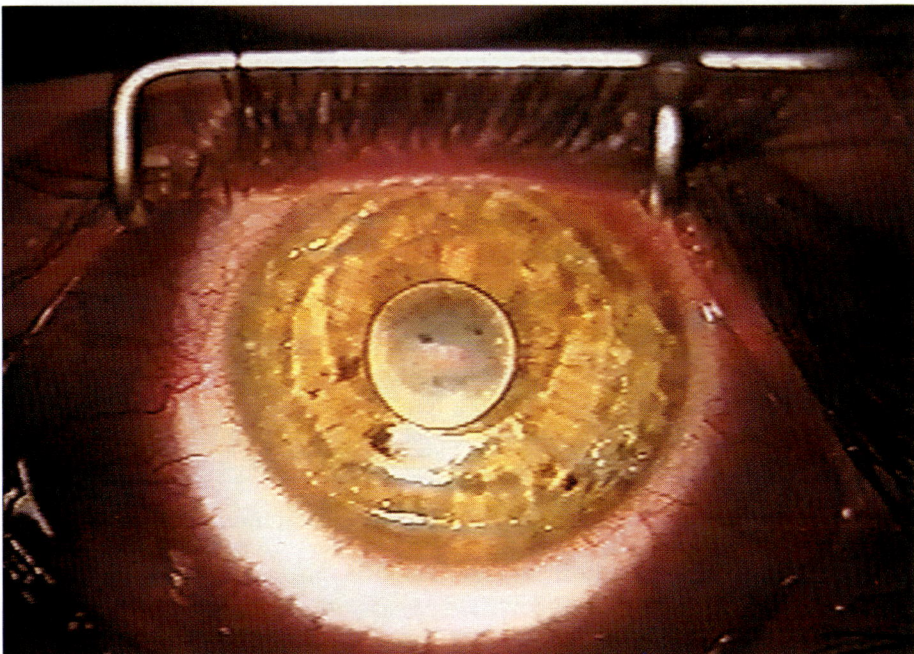

B

Figure 6–8. Technique of "Hyperopic PTK" (see also Fig. 3–26). **(A)** Following a 6.5 mm PTK directly applied to the center of the cornea, a sterile soft contact lens has been trephined to 4.0 mm and is placed with forceps over the center of the pupil. **(B)** As additional laser ablation is applied, the contact lens mask absorbs the central beam, preventing additional ablation to the central 4.0 mm of the cornea. *(Continued on following page)*

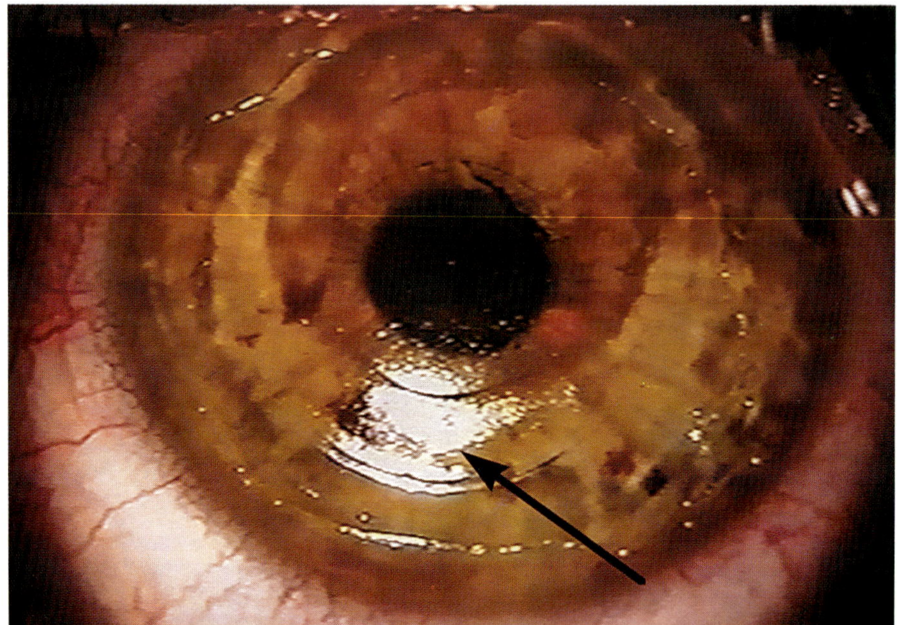

C

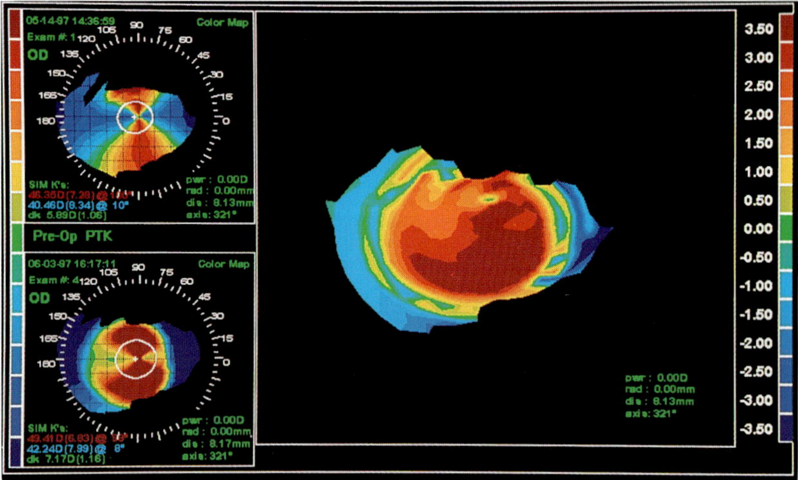

D

Figure 6–8 (cont.) (**C**) This creates a deeper annulus, or gutter, at the periphery of the ablation (arrow), leading to mitigation of corneal flattening induced by the large area ablation. (**D**) Postoperative differential topography map shows actual mild steepening of the central cornea following PTK in a previously hyperopic patient.

Case 27

HISTORY AND PREOPERATIVE EVALUATION

A 28-year-old woman with recurrent Reis-Buckler's corneal dystrophy presented with a spectacle-corrected visual acuity of 20/100 (Fig. 6–9). She had undergone PTK 2 years earlier using the standard polishing technique with 427 pulses at a 5.0 mm beam diameter and a smoothing annulus of 100 pulses at 2.0 mm. Despite the peripheral annulus of treatment, a 4 diopter hyperopic shift resulted. Spherical equivalent refraction was +3.50 diopters.

SURGICAL THERAPY AND OUTCOME

Given the hyperopic shift caused by the first PTK, a transepithelial technique with adjunctive "hyperopic" correction was used. A 6.5 mm beam diameter was chosen and the laser was directly applied to the central cornea. Two hundred pulses were used to remove the epithelium; epithelial removal was monitored by observing the blue fluorescence and its disappearance. An additional 100 pulses were used to clear the superficial opacity. The central area, measuring approximately 5.0 mm was then masked with methylcellulose 2.5%, and an additional 100 pulses was applied to create a "hyperopic" correction (Fig. 3–26). Following the procedure, the central cornea was

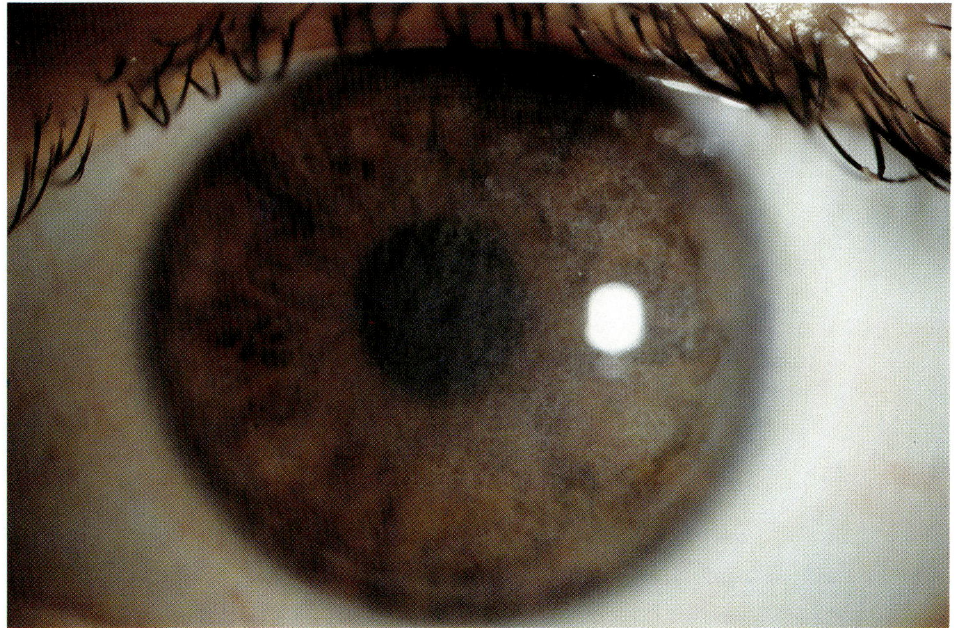

Figure 6–9. Case 27. **(A)** Preoperative appearance of a 28-year-old woman with recurrent Reis-Buckler's corneal dystrophy. Visual acuity is 20/100 with a spherical equivalent refraction of +3.50 diopters. *(Continued on following page)*

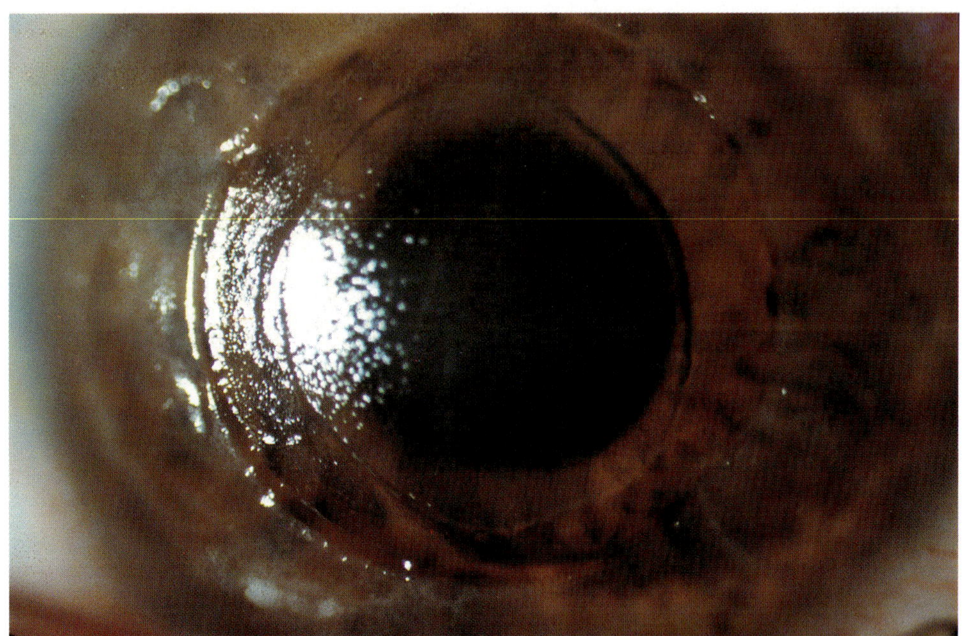

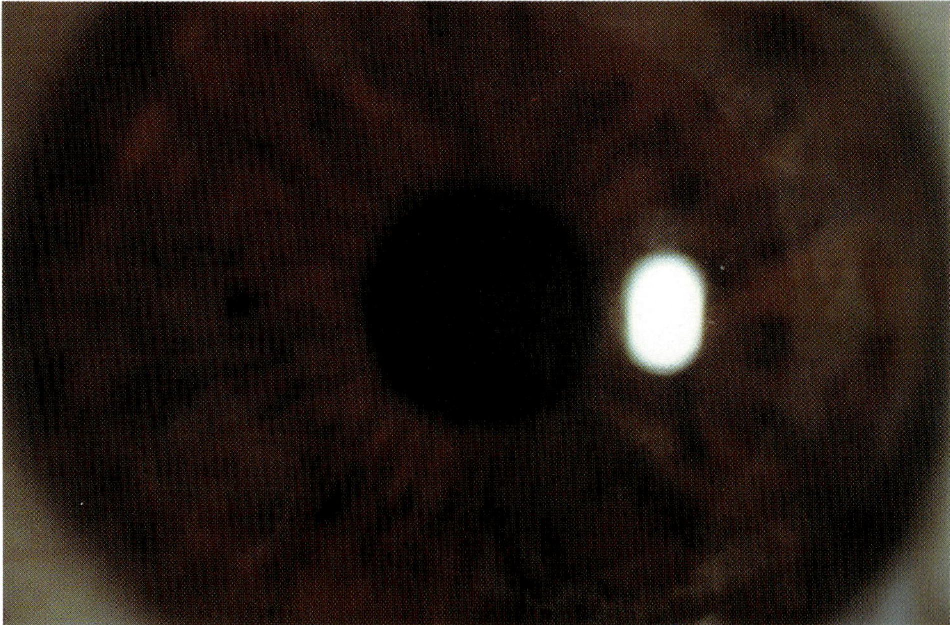

Figure 6–9 (B). Immediately following treatment using a direct laser application via a transepithelial technique and masking of the central cornea to create a "hyperopic" correction, the cornea is clearer and the annulus of additional "hyperopic" treatment is clearly seen. **(C)** At 2 weeks postoperatively, the central cornea is much clearer and visual acuity has improved to 20/40 with a spherical equivalent refraction of +3.00 diopters.

clearer and visual acuity had improved to 20/40 with a spherical equivalent refraction of +3.0 diopters. Thus, compared with her previous treatment outcome, hyperopic shifting was mitigated using this technique.

Case 28

HISTORY AND PREOPERATIVE EVALUATION

A 64-year-old man presented with a superficial corneal scar following multiple pterygium excisions (Fig. 6–10). Visual acuity was 20/100 with a spherical equivalent refraction of +6.0 diopters. Thus, compared with her previous treatment outcome, hyperopic shifting was mitigated using this technique.

SURGICAL THERAPY AND OUTCOME

A transepithelial approach with adjunctive "hyperopic" correction was chosen as in the previous case. A 6.5 mm beam was used to remove the scar. The central cornea was then masked with methylcellulose 2.5% and additional pulses at 6.5 mm were used to create a peripheral annulus measuring approximately 1 mm in diameter. During this procedure, methylcellulose 2.5% was reapplied carefully if it flowed from its position on the center of the cornea. Postoperatively, visual acuity improved to 20/30, and refraction remained stable at +6.0 diopters.

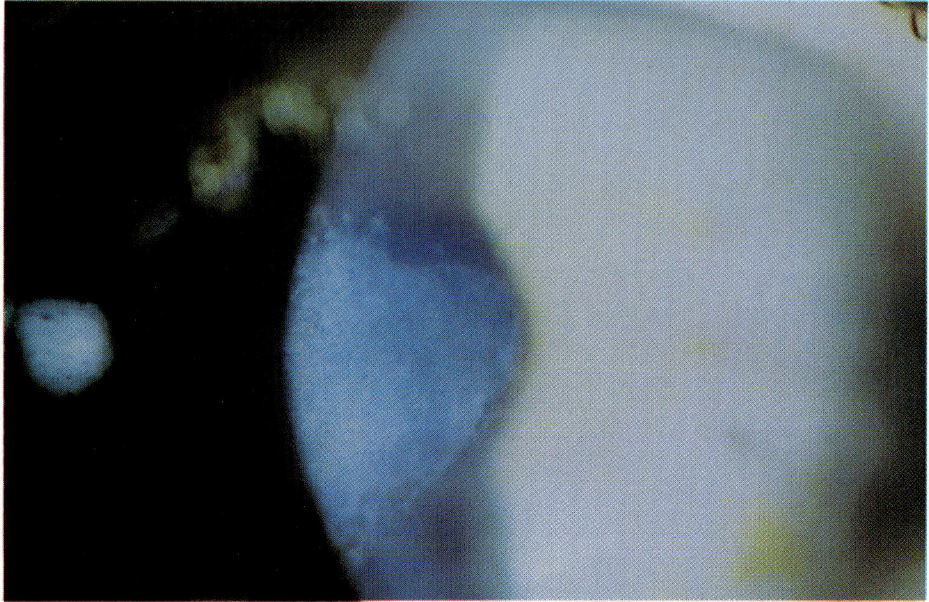

A

Figure 6–10. Case 28. **(A)** A 64-year-old man presented with a superficial corneal scar following multiple pterygium excisions. Visual acuity is 20/100 with a spherical equivalent refraction of +6.0 diopters. *(Continued on following page)*

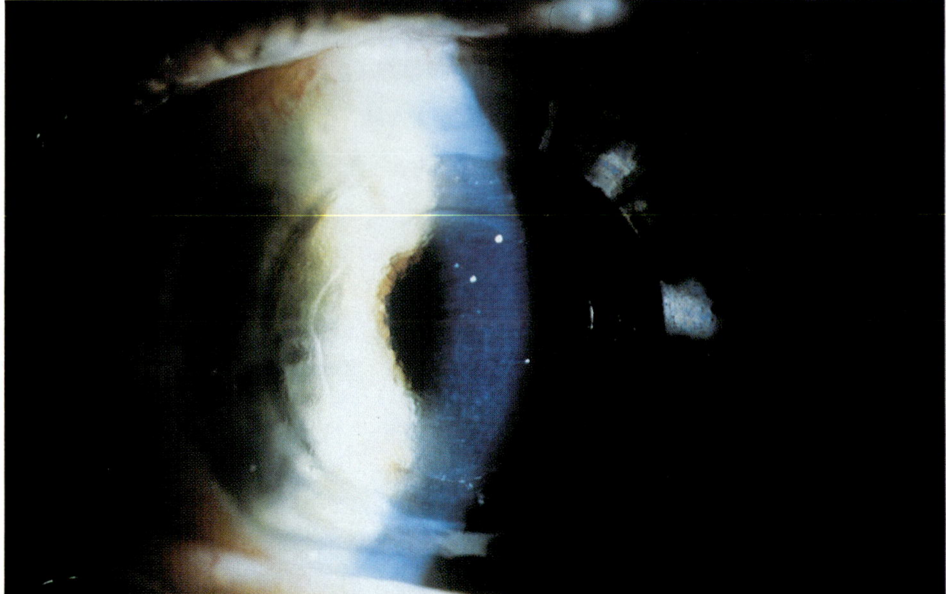

B

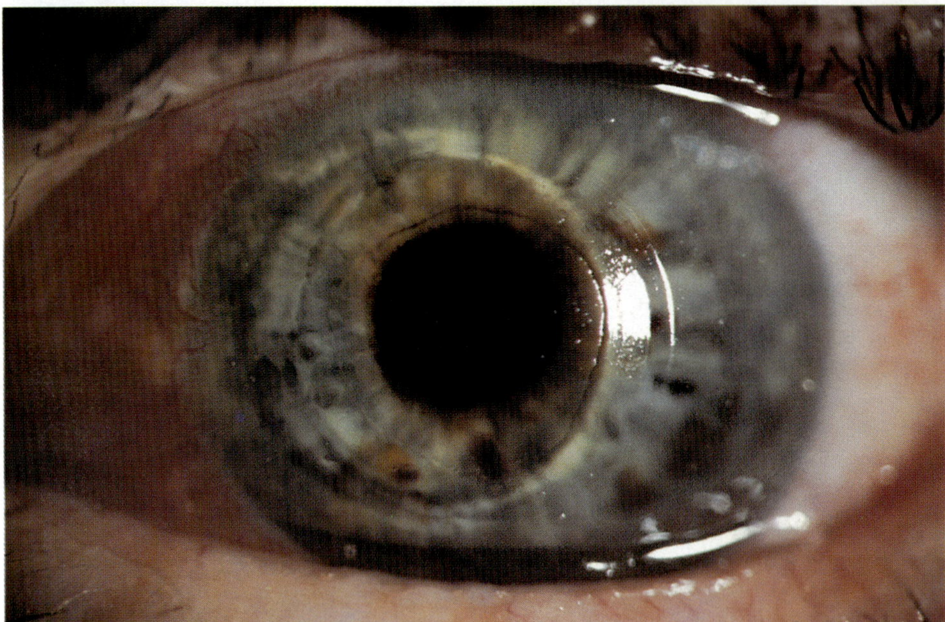

C

Figure 6–10 (B,C).   Immediately following treatment using a direct laser application via a transepithelial technique and masking of the central cornea to create a "hyperopic" correction, the cornea is clear, and the annulus of additional "hyperopic" treatment is clearly seen. Visual acuity improved to 20/30, and refraction remained stable at +6.0 diopters.

Treating Refractive Shifts and Topography Changes

Undesirable refractive shifts and topographic changes may lead to poor vision and anisometropia after PTK. In some cases, correction at the corneal plane with either soft or rigid contact lenses is helpful. In the case of abnormal topography, a rigid lens is preferred. In some cases, retreatment may be performed. In such cases an attempt is made to treat steep areas of the cornea in a focal manner (Fig. 6–11, Case 29).[1] Such an approach must be used with caution, however. Preoperatively, it must be determined whether or not a steep area represents an elevation or a depression. This may be ascertained by clinical examination, ultrasonic pachymetry, contact lens fit, and videokeratography units that accurately measure surface evaluation. Steep areas that are depressed should not have further tissue removed.

Conclusions

A perfect scar removal with a clear postoperative cornea may be complicated by unwanted refractive shifts. Patients, therefore, should be made aware of both the potential for refractive change and the alternatives, such as rigid contact lenses,[13] available to correct vision postoperatively after PTK. For

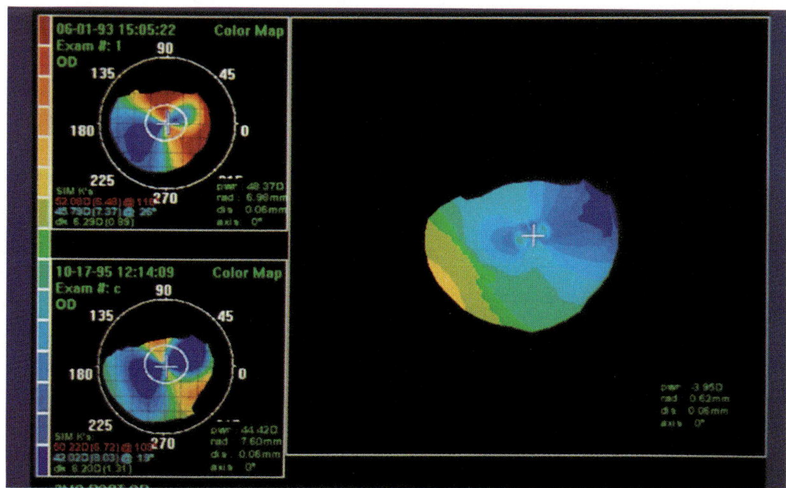

Figure 6–11.   Case 29. Following initial PTK for a recurrent dystrophy in a corneal graft, irregular astigmatism has developed **(Top Left)**. Focal treatment of the steep areas with the excimer laser (453 pulses at 5.0 mm and 285 pulses at 4.0 mm) has smoothed the corneal contours, leaving regular astigmatism amenable to spectacle correction **(Bottom Left)**. A differential topography map **(Right)** shows desired flattening of the steep areas.

instance, removal of a central corneal scar may improve best-corrected spectacle or rigid contact lens visual acuity but actually decrease uncorrected visual acuity as a result of either a refractive shift away from emmetropia or induced irregular astigmatism. Central corneal smoothing in a myopic patient may be rewarded with both a clearer cornea and reduced refractive error while central scar removal in a hyperopic patient, while clearing the cornea, may result in unacceptable hyperopia and perturbation of the corneal topography.

Proper case selection and surgical planning thus are essential to obtaining a successful result of the PTK procedure. Patients most suited to PTK appear to be those with surface excrescences where the procedure will both clear the cornea and improve the corneal surface optical contour. The surgeon and patient must understand the goals of the procedure, and a meticulously planned surgical strategy should be directed at the specific corneal disorder. Such preparation and execution will best lead to a satisfactory postoperative clinical result.

References

1. Gibralter R, Trokel SL. Correction of irregular astigmatism with the excimer laser. Ophthalmology 1994;101:1310–1315.
2. Hersh PS, Burnstein Y, Carr J, Etwaru G, Mayers M. Phototherapeutic keratectomy: surgical strategies and clinical outcomes. Ophthalmology 1996;103:1210–1222.
3. Maloney RK, Thompson V, Ghiselli G, Durrie D, Waring GO, O'Connell M. A prospective multicenter trial of excimer laser phototherapeutic keratectomy for corneal vision loss. Am J Ophthalmol 1996;122:149–160.
4. Campos M, Nielsen S, Szerenyi K, Garbus JJ, McDonnell PJ. Clinical follow-up of phototherapeutic keratectomy for the treatment of corneal opacities. Am J Ophthalmol 1993;115:433–440.
5. Sher N, Bowers RA, Zabel RW, Frantz JM, Eifferman RA, Brown DC, Rowsey JJ, Parker P, Chen V, Lindstrom RL. Clinical use of the 193-nm excimer laser in the treatment of corneal scars. Arch Ophthalmol 1991;109:491–498.
6. Wu WCS, Stark WJ, Green WR. Corneal wound healing excimer laser keratectomy. Arch Ophthalmol 1991;109:1426–1432.
7. Simon G, Ren Q, Kervick GN, Parel JM. Optics of the corneal epithelium. J Refract Corneal Surg 1993;9:42–50.
8. Hersh PS, Carr JD. Excimer laser photorefractive keratectomy. Ophthalmic Practice 1995;13:126–133.
9. Kornmehl EW, Steinert RF, Puliafito CA. A comparative study of masking fluids for excimer laser phototherapeutic keratectomy. Arch Ophthalmol 1991;109:860–863.
10. Blaker JW, Hersh PS. Theoretical and clinical effect of corneal curvature on excimer laser photorefractive keratectomy. Refract Corneal Surg 1994;10:571–574.
11. Gartry D, Kerr Muir M, Marshall J. Excimer laser treatment of corneal surface pathology: a laboratory and clinical study. Br J Ophthalmol 1991;75:258–267.
12. McDonnell P, Seiler T. Phototherapeutic keratectomy with excimer laser for Reis-Buckler's corneal dystrophy. J Refract Corneal Surg 1992;8:306–310.
13. Eggink FAGJ, Beekhuis WH. Granular dystrophy of the cornea. Contact lens fitting after phototherapeutic keratectomy. Cornea 1995;14:217–222.

Phototherapeutic Keratectomy for Complications of Excimer Laser Refractive Surgery

Techniques of phototherapeutic keratectomy, in addition to treating corneal pathology, can be used to correct a variety of complications of excimer laser photorefractive keratectomy.[1–13] This is an extensive subject itself; thus, the goal of this chapter is simply to introduce general concepts in such treatments.

Indications

There are two general indications for PTK following PRK:

Corneal haze and scarring. Substantial corneal haze or scarring resulting from aggressive wound healing after PRK may lead to regression of effect and loss of best corrected visual acuity, as well as optical side effects such as decreased contrast sensitivity, monocular diplopia, glare, and halo.[14–16] Most studies have shown corneal haze to decrease with time following the procedure.[13,17] In some cases of recalcitrant scarring, however, PTK may be used to clear the opacity.[18–20]

Corneal topography abnormalities. Irregularities in the postoperative PRK corneal topography, such as central islands and keyhole patterns, may degrade the patient's spectacle corrected visual acuity and cause subjective optical sequelae such as glare, halo, and monocular diplopia.[21–30] In properly selected cases, use of PTK may help to smooth the surface topography and correct such side effects.

Treatment of Corneal Haze and Scars Following Photorefractive Keratectomy

The general considerations of PTK for the treatment of corneal scars and opacities pertain to the post-PRK cornea. The depth of the scar, its contour (i.e., elevated or depressed), location, and initial refractive error all must be considered to achieve a successful result. Such findings will suggest the appropriate surgical strategy.

CASE 30

History and preoperative evaluation. A 48-year-old man with a refraction of −8.50–0.25 × 15 in the right eye had undergone a 12-incision radial keratotomy. Two years later, he underwent PRK for residual myopia of −5.00–1.00 × 150. Photorefractive keratectomy was performed using a 5.0 mm ablation zone. Following PRK, he achieved 20/30 uncorrected visual acuity, but complained of glare as well as monocular diplopia in the right eye which was more severe at night.[30] Such symptoms were not present before the laser treatment.

Slit-lamp examination 18 months following PRK revealed a ring of moderate (2 + on a scale of 0 to 4 +) subepithelial haze, approximately 4 to 5 mm in diameter with a relatively clear cornea and an iron line centrally (Fig. 7-1A). Best spectacle corrected vision was 20/20 with refraction of +1.25–2.00 × 180. A standard corneal videokeratography map showed a smooth, toric-with-axis pattern[21] with good centration and no irregularities (Fig. 7-1B).[31–33]

There was decreased contrast sensitivity at all spatial frequencies. Pupillary diameter measured 7 mm in the light and 9 mm under low light normal conditions. The patient, a doctoral candidate, stated that his diplopia improved somewhat with 1% pilocarpine drops. In addition, trial of a rigid contact lens only partially ameliorated his diplopia symptoms, indicating scarring rather than irregular astigmatism as the primary etiology of his symptoms.

Surgical therapy and outcome. After the patient received informed consent, with the potential of a hyperopic refractive shift carefully explained, a transepithelial PTK was performed. The transepithelial technique was chosen, since the surface of the cornea appeared smooth and lustrous. Epithelial removal was monitored by observing the blue fluorescence of the ablating epithelium. Using a 6.5 mm beam diameter, approximately 200 pulses were necessary to remove the epithelium. One hundred four additional pulses were then delivered, again at 6.5 mm, to remove the scar. Scar removal was monitored by slit lamp examination.

Postoperatively, spectacle-corrected vision remained 20/20, with refraction of +0.25–1.75 × 170. The corneal scar was substantially cleared and monocular diplopia had resolved, allowing the patient to read comfortably with his reading correction.

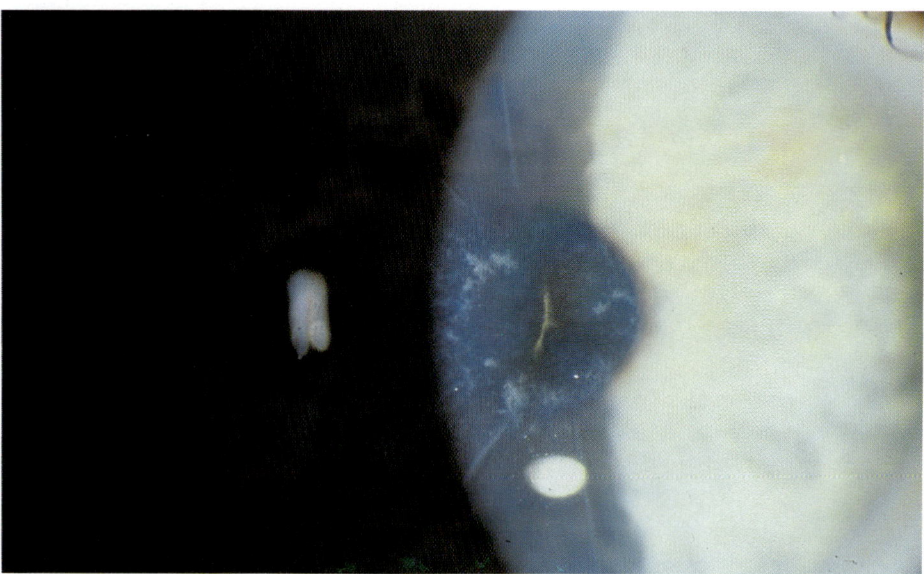

A

Figure 7-1.   Case 30. **(A)** Slit lamp appearance of 48-year-old man 3 years following 12 incision radial keratotomy and 18 months following photorefractive keratectomy for residual myopia. Note radial keratotomy incisions, ring of subepithelial corneal haze, and central iron line. Best spectacle corrected vision was 20/20, but patient complained of monocular diplopia and glare symptoms. **(B)** A videokeratography map showed a regular, toric-with-axis pattern with good centration and no irregularities. **(C)** Following PTK (transepithelial technique, 6.5 mm beam diameter, 304 pulses), the cornea has cleared, spectacle corrected visual acuity is 20/20, and monocular diplopia has improved. (Figures 7-1A and B reprinted with permission from Hersh et al.[34]) (*Continued on following page*)

Discussion. This patient's main complaint was monocular diplopia during reading. The goal was to give good reading vision, and the patient understood that PTK might increase his need for reading glasses. Again, this case demonstrates that preoperative identification of the individual patient's postoperative goal is important in planning the PTK procedure. In this case, there was little hyperopic shift; however, a prior understanding of possible refractive changes and the need for postoperative spectacle correction is necessary, especially in patients who are being treated for complications of refractive surgery where their initial goal was to decrease dependency on glasses and contact lenses.

CASE 31

History and preoperative evaluation. A 37-year-old male myope presented with a refraction of -5.25D OD and $-5.00-0.50 \times 170$ OS correcting visual acuity to 20/20 in both eyes, respectively. The patient underwent PRK to the left eye with an attempted correction of -5.3 D. Surgery was uncomplicated.

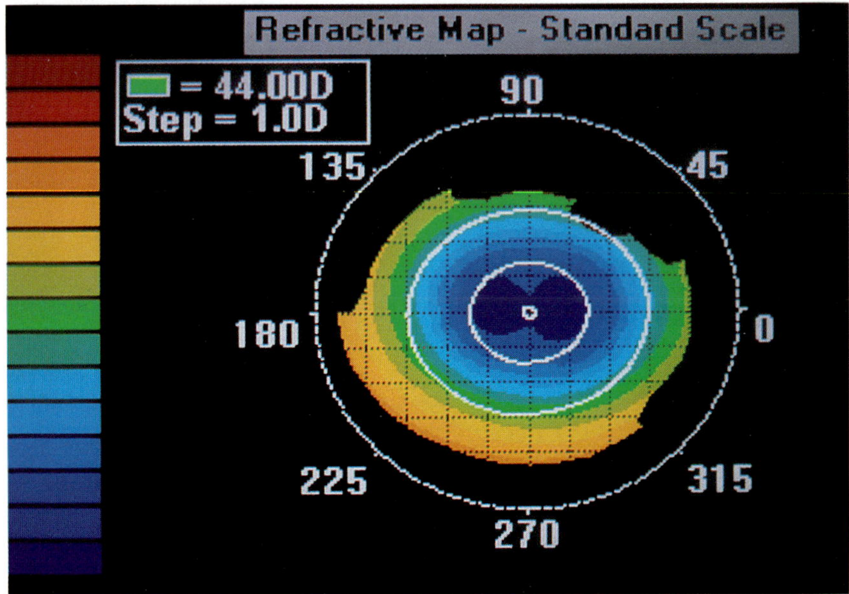

Figure 7–1 (B)

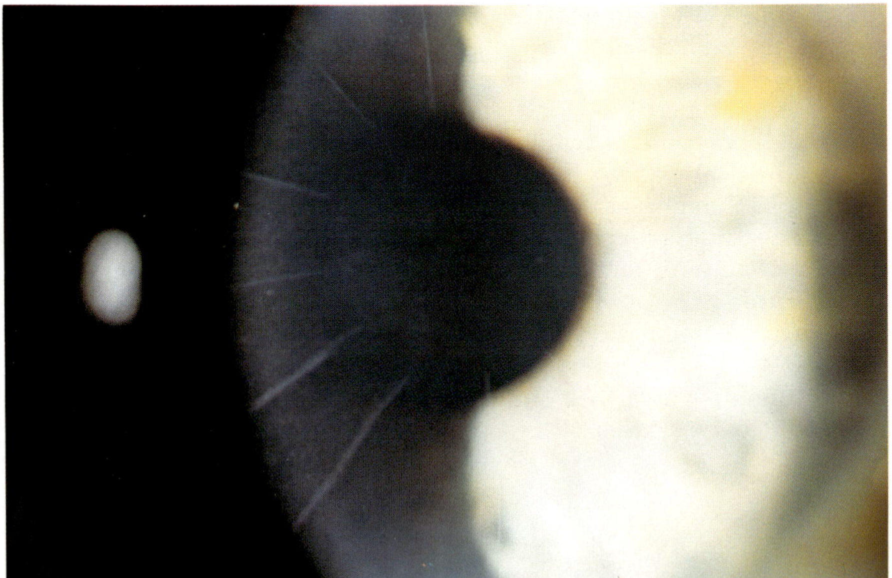

Figure 7–1 (C)

The clinical course is summarized in Table 7-1. When seen at the 1-month postoperative visit, refraction was plano-1.00 × 180 correcting acuity to 20/16. Slit lamp examination showed a 5 mm area of trace haze (Fig. 7-2A). Videokeratography showed a regular central flattening of the corneal topography (Fig. 7-2B). Fluoromethalone eye drops were reduced from 4 to 3 times daily. Examination at 2 months following PRK showed an increase in haze grade to mild, but refraction and best corrected vision were unchanged. The fluoromethalone drops were tapered to twice daily for 2 weeks, once a day for 1 week, and every other day for a further week then discontinued.

At 3 months following PRK, mild myopic regression was seen with −0.75–0.75 × 150 correcting visual acuity to 20/20. Haze was still graded as mild for the central 5 mm of the cornea (Fig. 7-2C). Fluoromethalone and diclofenac eye drops were started (4 times daily for 1 week, twice daily for 1 week, once a week, and then discontinued) for treatment of the haze. At 6 months postoperatively, haze had increased to moderate (Fig. 7-2D).[34] Refraction was −3.00–1.50 × 145 giving 20/32 visual acuity. Corneal videokeratography showed a localized steepening over the area of the scar formation (Fig. 7-2E).[35] The patient described glare and halo symptoms which he subjectively graded as 2 for glare and 1 for halo (scale from 0 to 4). In view of the increased haze and regression, fluoromethalone and diclofenac eye drops were again prescribed 4 times daily. Follow-up at 8 months showed the same degree of haze with a refraction of −3.50–1.50 × 150, which corrected visual acuity to 20/32. Glare and halo symptoms were unchanged.

Surgical therapy and outcome. Having failed medical therapy, mechanical superficial keratectomy (SK) and excimer laser retreatment were two options considered to remove the haze and reduce the myopia. Given the focal plaquelike appearance of the haze, the patient underwent superficial keratectomy.[36,37] The epithelium was carefully removed with blunt dissection using cellulose sponges and the edge of a rounded microsurgical blade. The superficial scar tissue was then meticulously peeled with dry cellulose sponges, 0.12 mm forceps, and the blade. Care was taken to remain in a cleavage plane between the scar tissue and normal corneal stroma. Upon completion of the procedure, the bed appeared smooth, and little changed from its appearance immediately following initial PRK (Fig. 7-2F). A combined antibiotic/corticosteroid ointment and a pressure patch were applied and the patient followed daily until epithelialization occurred on the third postoperative day.

Two weeks after superficial keratectomy, uncorrected visual acuity was 20/50 in the left eye. Refraction was −0.75–0.75 × 90 producing 20/32 visual acuity with a 5mm central zone of trace reticular haze. The postoperative fluoromethalone eye drops were slowly tapered over 3 months. Three months following SK, refraction was −1.75D correcting vision to 20/20. A

Table 7-1.   Case 31: Clinical Course*

	PRE-OP	POSTOP MONTH # AFTER 1ST PRK					SK†	MONTH # AFTER SK		PRK #2	MONTH # AFTER REPEAT PRK		
		1	2	3	6	9		3	6		1	2	3
Haze‡	0	1	2	2	4	4		2	4		1	1	1
Glare‡	0	0	0	0	2	1		3	2		1	1	1
Halo‡	0	0	0	0	0	0		2	2		1	1	1
Sphere (D)	−5.00	0	0	−0.75	−3.00	−3.00		−1.75	−3.5		0	−0.5	−0.5
Cyl (D)	−0.50	−1.00	−0.75	−0.75	−1.5	−1.25		0	−1		0	−0.5	−0.25
Axis	170	180	90	150	150	145			155			180	180
UCVA (20/x)	20	20	32	25	100	160		50	200		25	25	25
BCVA (20/x)	20	16	20	20	25	32		20	32		25	25	25

Reprinted with permission from Carr et al.[18]
*Table courtesy of Jonathan Carr, M.D.
†SK = superficial keratectomy
‡Subjective patient questionnaire results; scale 0 to 4

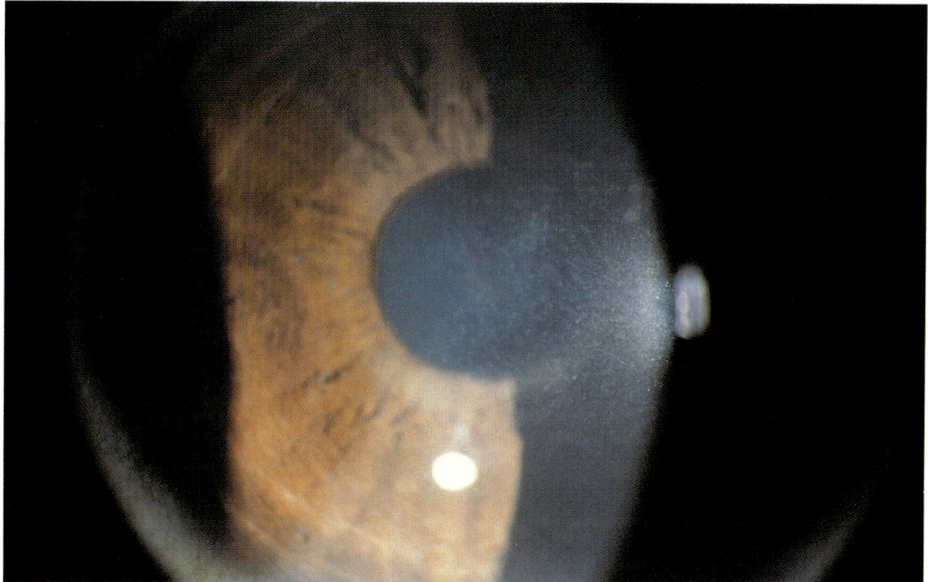

A

Figure 7-2.   Case 31. **(A)** One month following PRK, attempted correction 5.3 diopter. Trace central corneal haze can be seen. *(Continued on following five pages)*

mild haze was noted. At 4 months following SK, the refraction continued to regress to −3.00D producing 20/20 acuity with mild haze still noted (Fig. 7-2G). At 8 months following SK, the refraction had regressed to −3.50–1.00 × 155 correcting visual acuity to 20/32. Corneal haze was graded as moderate (Fig. 7-2H). Given the poor success of superficial keratectomy, a repeat excimer laser procedure was performed with an attempted correction of 3.50D, with the dual goal of removing the corneal scar and achieving refractive correction. The epithelium was removed using a 6.5 mm PTK of 182 pulses, monitored by epithelial fluorescence. Epithelial removal was stopped when a confluent black ring of nonfluorescence was noted around the central treatment zone, indicating that the laser ablation had reached the stroma peripherally. At this point, the excimer PRK was then carried out without complication using a 6.0mm ablation zone (Fig. 7-2I).

Postoperatively, the patient was treated vigorously with corticosteroids starting with a prednisolone acetate 1% every 2 hours and tapering over a period of many months. Examination 1 month later showed a plano refraction and spectacle corrected visual acuity of 20/25; glare and halo symptoms had decreased. Three months after the excimer retreatment, uncorrected visual acuity was 20/25. Refraction was −0.50–0.25 × 180. Glare and halo were still subjectively rated as a score of 1 and trace haze was confined to a small area temporal to the visual axis. Videokeratography showed a restoration of the regular central flattening of the cornea (Fig. 7-2J). One year

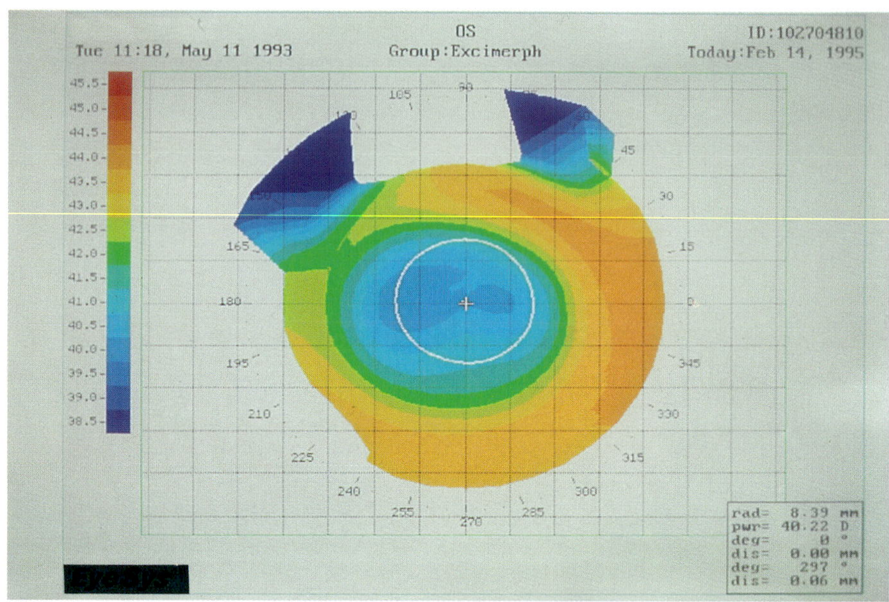

B

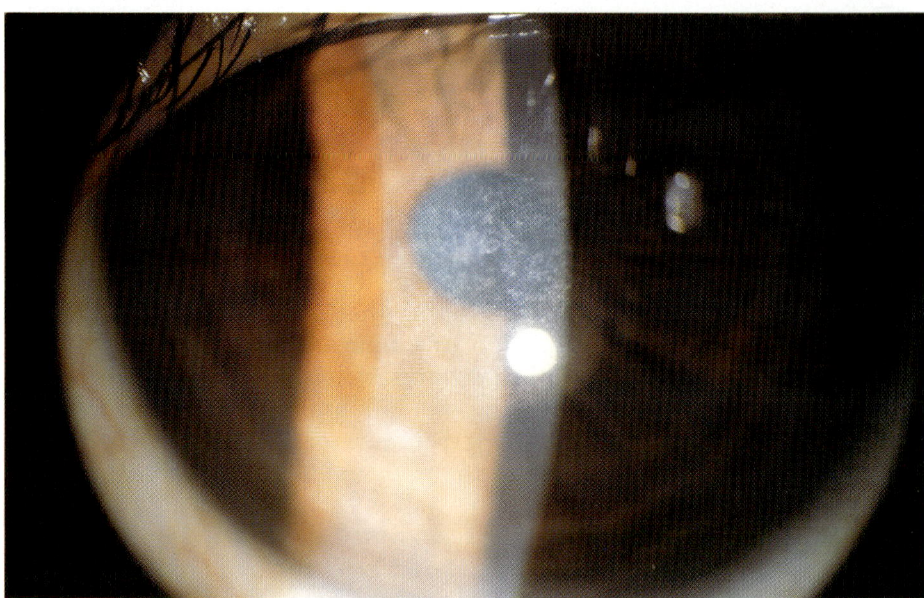

C

Figure 7-2. **(B)** Videokeratography map 1 month following PRK. The central cornea shows a centered ablation with a regular pattern. **(C)** Three months postoperatively; mild central haze can be seen.

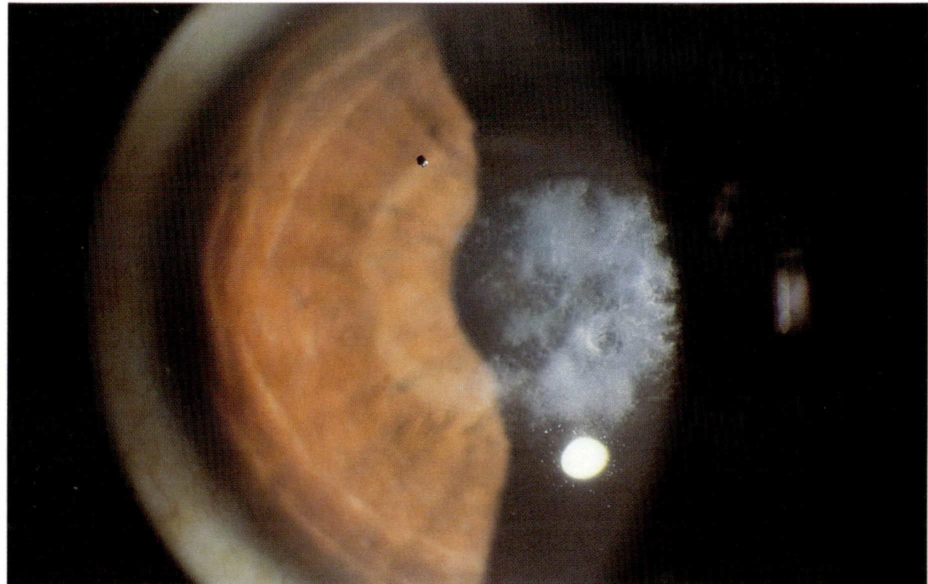

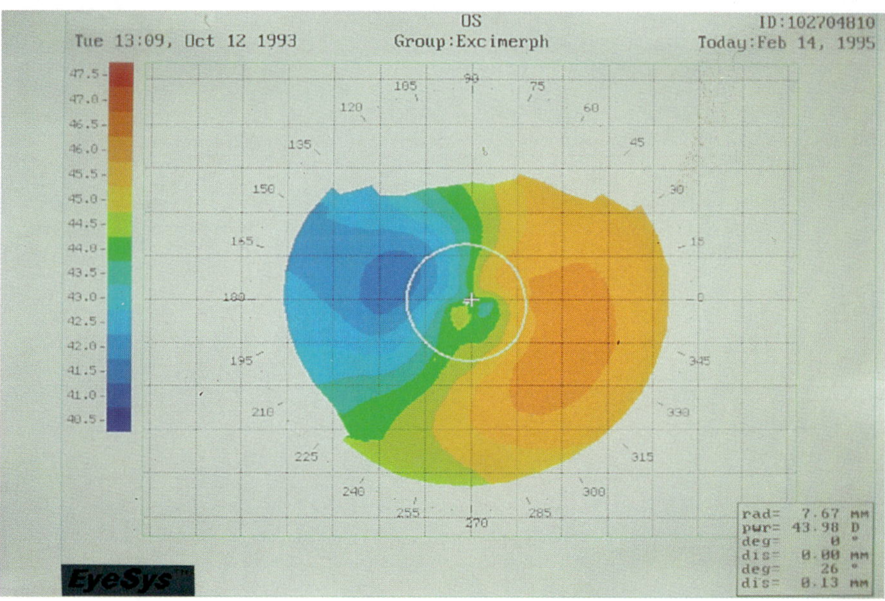

Figure 7-2. **(D)** Six months postoperatively; a reticular subepithelial fibrous plaque has formed. **(E)** Videokeratography map showing steepening overlying the area of corneal scar formation.

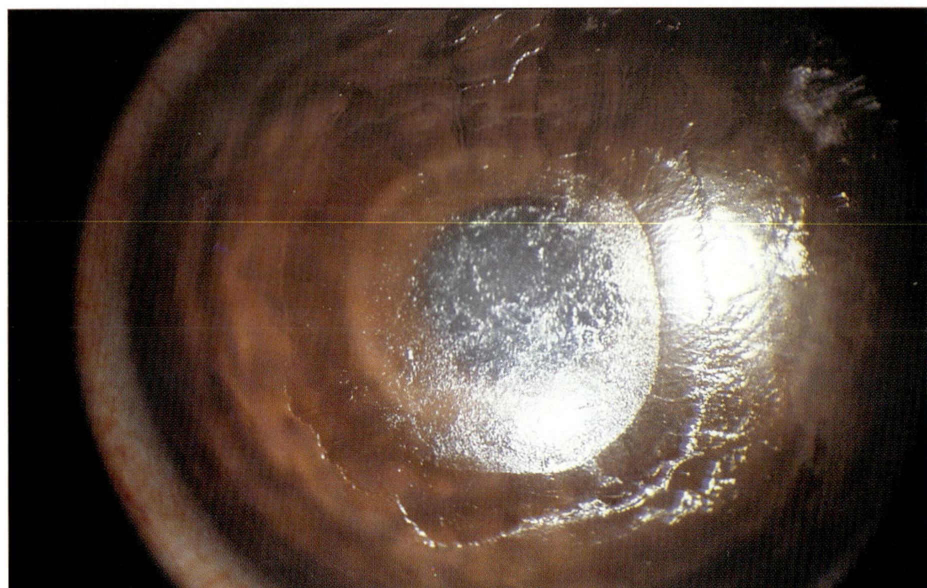

F

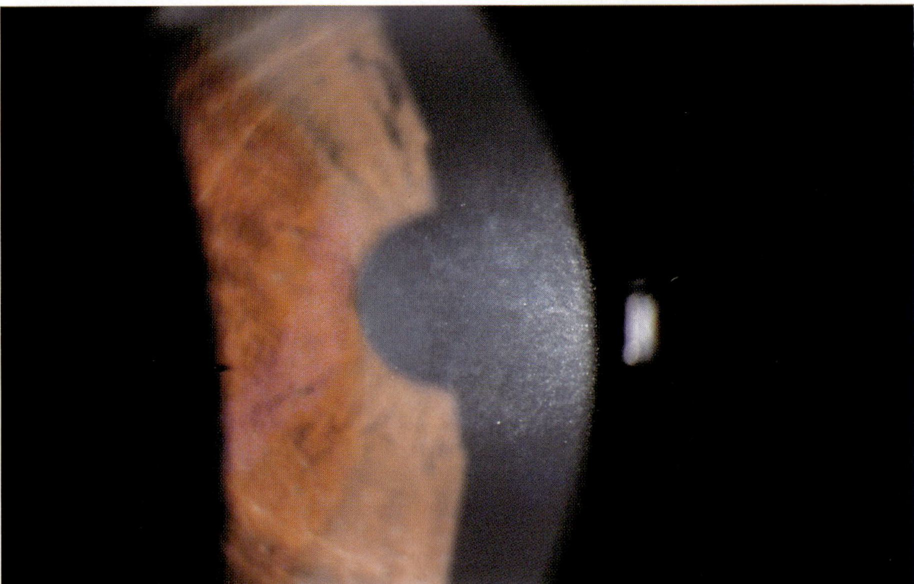

G

Figure 7-2. **(F)** Cornea immediately following superficial keratectomy, showing a clear stromal bed with no evidence of scar tissue. Note distinct edges of the original ablation zone. **(G)** Four months following superficial keratectomy, mild haze can be seen centrally.

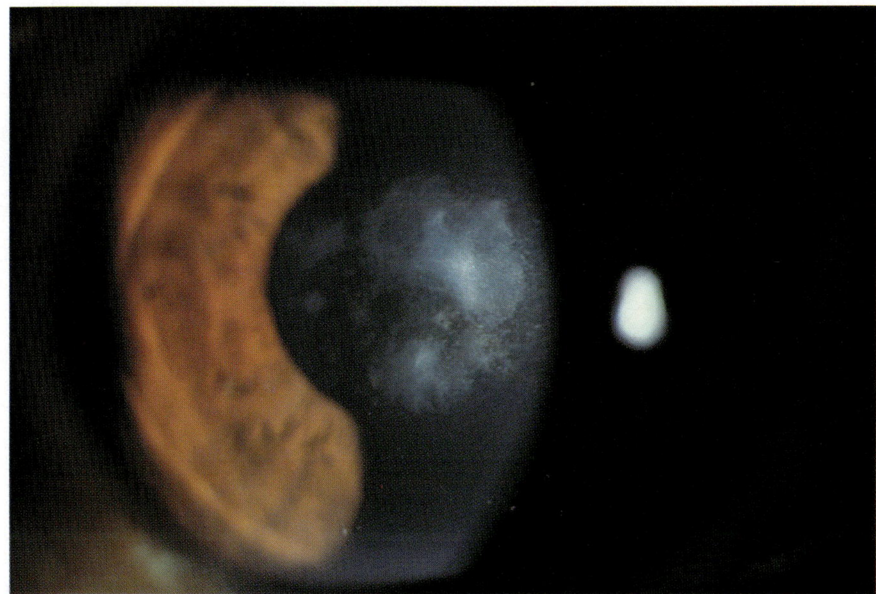

Figure 7-2. **(H)** Eight months following superficial keratectomy, showing reposition of a fibrous plaque. **(I)** Cornea immediately following repeated excimer PRK. The central cornea is clear, with no evidence of haze.

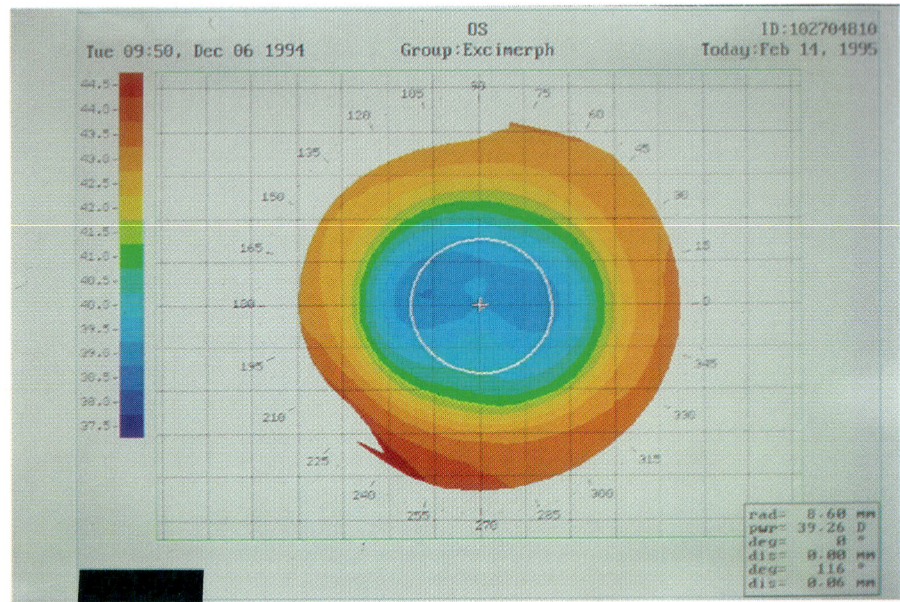

J

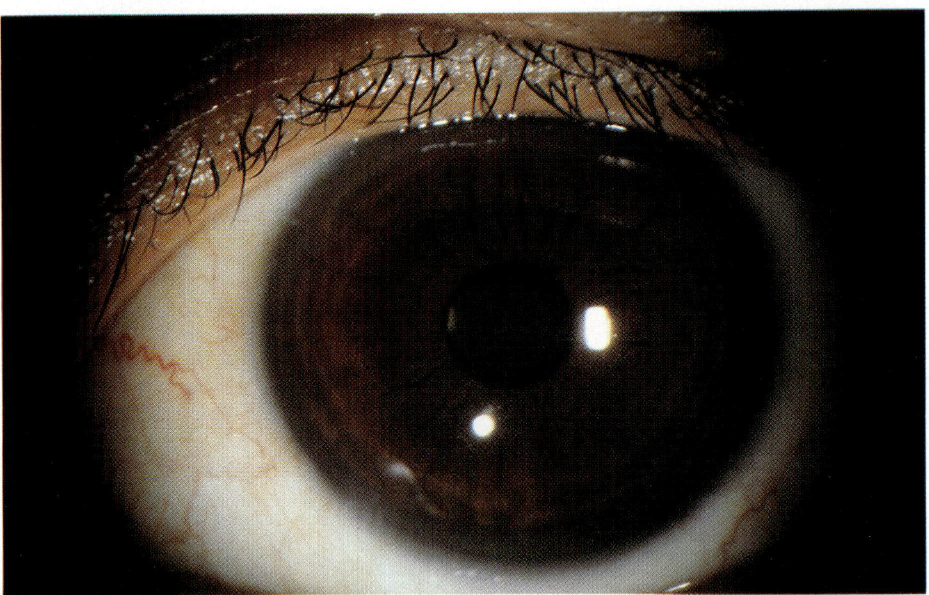

K

Figure 7-2. **(J)** Videokeratography map shows restoration of a smooth topography pattern. **(K)** Six months postoperatively, the cornea remains clear. (Reprinted with permission from Carr et al.[18])

postoperatively, the cornea remained clear with 20/25 uncorrected visual acuity and 20/20 spectacle corrected visual acuity (Fig. 7-2K).

Discussion. In this patient, topical fluoromethalone and diclofenac medications were started at the 6-month postoperative visit at a time when haze and myopic regression had become a significant problem. This treatment, however, had no detectable effect on either haze or refractive error. Thus, superficial keratectomy was undertaken. The procedure has been previously described[37] as a way of removing scar tissue forming as a result of excimer laser PRK. These authors make the point that the superficial keratectomy compares reasonably with the published results of excimer laser retreatments and that superficial keratectomy does not preclude further excimer treatments. As seen in this patient, moreover, the specific haze morphology—interposition of plaquelike fibrous tissue between the epithelium and normal clear stroma—actually seemed to make mechanical superficial keratectomy the preferred procedure, since the plaque could be stripped off, leaving the ablation bed after SK much as it had appeared after the original PRK. This may be in contrast to other patients demonstrating haze, where the fibrous deposition is actually intercalated with the corneal stroma.

Superficial keratectomy in this patient improved the best corrected visual acuity in the postoperative period and also reduced glare and halo side effects. There was also a reduction in the myopic refractive error with consequently improved uncorrected visual acuity. However, regression and haze recurred after 3 months, the etiology of which is unclear. In this case, therefore, mechanical superficial keratectomy successfully removed the scar, yet was met with poor longer-term results and recrudescence of the fibrous plaque.

Subsequent transepithelial excimer laser treatment led to successful long-term results.[18] The reason for the relative success of the two procedures in this case are unclear. It has been suggested that transepithelial laser treatment will lead to less activation of corneal wound healing in the superficial stroma after excimer laser treatment compared with mechanical removal.[20] Likewise, laser ablation of the scar could have led to less subjacent stromal damage than mechanical scar removal.[19] Alternatively, the high postoperative corticosteroid dosage after the repeat excimer laser treatment may have led to decreased propensity to recurrent scarring.[38–41,50] Although the efficacy of corticosteroid treatment after standard photorefractive keratectomy has been questioned,[39–40] carefully supervised corticosteroid treatment in the setting of corneal scarring and PTK or mechanical superficial keratectomy is likely advisable.[41]

Treatment of Corneal Topography Irregularities Following Photorefractive Keratectomy

As for other corneal abnormalities, it is essential to carefully assess the corneal contour when devising a surgical strategy to correct topography abnormalities. Eight distinct patterns of corneal topography following PRK have been defined based on analysis of differential topography maps:[21,29]

1. *Homogeneous.* Shows a uniform and symmetric flattening, often with a smooth power change gradient with a progressively decreasing power change proceeding from the center to the periphery of the treatment zone (Fig. 7-3A).

2. *Toric-with-axis.* Shows a meridionally symmetric treatment zone with a greater induced flattening (toric bowtie) in the steep preoperative axis. The differential between flattening and steepening in the two orthogonal meridians should be >0.5 diopters. This pattern presumably would decrease the patient's corneal toricity (Fig. 7-3B).

3. *Toric-against-axis.* Shows a meridionally symmetric treatment zone with a greater induced flattening (toric bowtie) in the flat preoperative axis. The differential between flattening and steepening in the two orthogonal meridians should be >0.5 diopters. This pattern presumably would increase the patient's corneal toricity (Fig. 7-3C).

4. *Semicircular.* Shows a general foreshortening of the treatment zone effect in one meridian, quantitatively measuring >1.0 mm in size and >1.0 diopter of relatively less flattening compared with the meridian 180 degrees away (Fig. 7-3D).

5. *Keyhole.* Shows topographic regions, quantitatively measuring >1.0 mm in size and 1.0 diopter of relatively less flattening, extending in from the periphery of the ablation zone in one meridian. Unlike the semicircular pattern, the area of relatively less power decrease encompasses less than 180 degrees of the periphery and extends as an apparent involution of diminished power decrease into the treatment zone (Fig. 7-3E).

6. *Central island.* Shows a central area of relatively less flattening measuring >1.0 mm in diameter and >1.0 diopter in power, and not extending to the periphery. The central island is surrounded around its entire periphery by areas of greater power diminution (Fig. 7-3F).

7. *Irregularly irregular.* Shows generalized irregularities over the treatment zone, defined as more than one area measuring >0.5 mm and >0.5 D in power from other areas at the same radius from the treatment zone center, and not conforming to the specific criteria of the other patterns described (Fig. 7-3G).

8. *Focal topography variant.* Shows a generally homogeneous pattern with a single irregularity measuring <1.0 mm in size or <1.0 diopter in power. Although this is only slightly different from the homogeneous pattern, it is intended to determine if minor topography variations, not meeting the criteria of the other patterns, affect clinical outcomes. This pattern has not been found to have clinical implications in past investigations (Fig. 7-3H).[21,30]

Treatment of such topography patterns is dictated by patient symptoms. Irregularities of the optical surface of the cornea, in particular central islands and keyholes, may lead to patient complaints of glare, halo, and monocular diplopia.[26] Of great importance when assessing topography maps and pat-

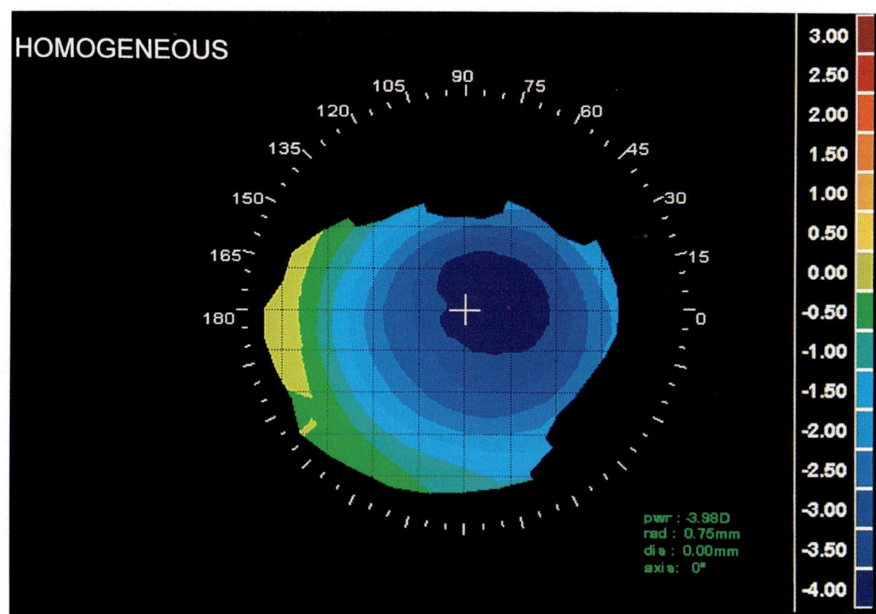

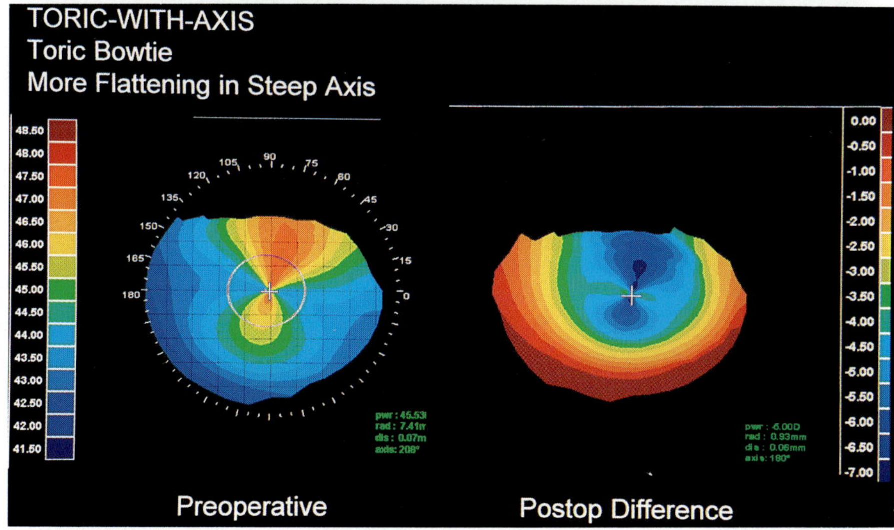

Figure 7-3.　Corneal topography patterns after PRK. **(A)** Homogeneous. **(B)** Toric-with-axis. *(Continued on following three pages)*

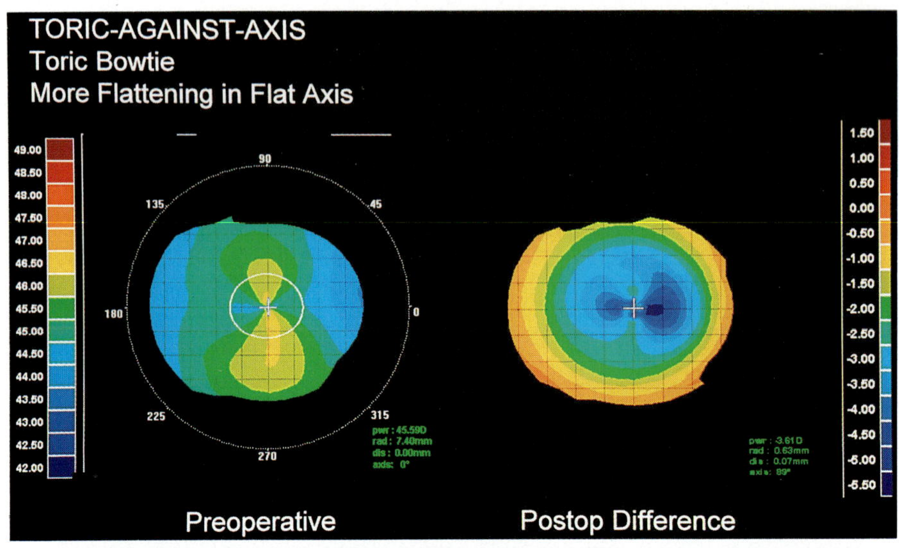

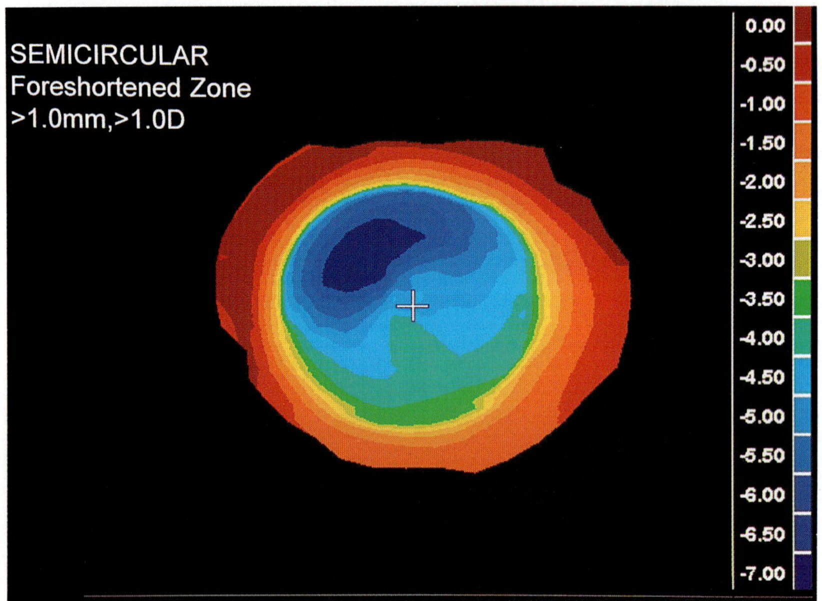

Figure 7-3. *Continued*   **(C)** Toric-against-axis. **(D)** Semicircular.

terns for potential laser treatment is the requirement to differentiate corneal curvature from corneal shape. While a steeply curved area on the topography map may indeed represent an actual elevation that will be improved by tissue removal with PTK, it may conversely represent a more rapid falling off or depressed area, which would be exacerbated by tissue removal

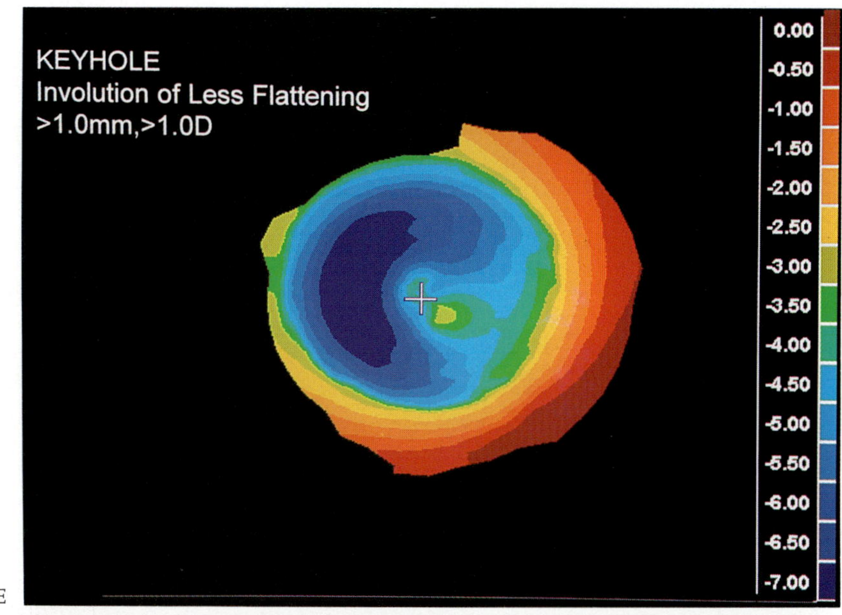

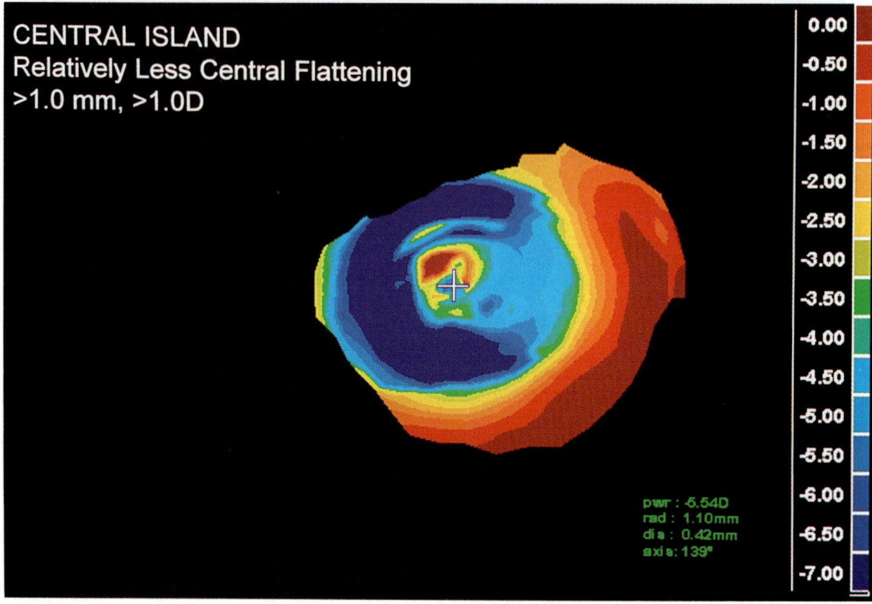

Figure 7-3. *Continued*   **(E)** Keyhole. **(F)** Central island.

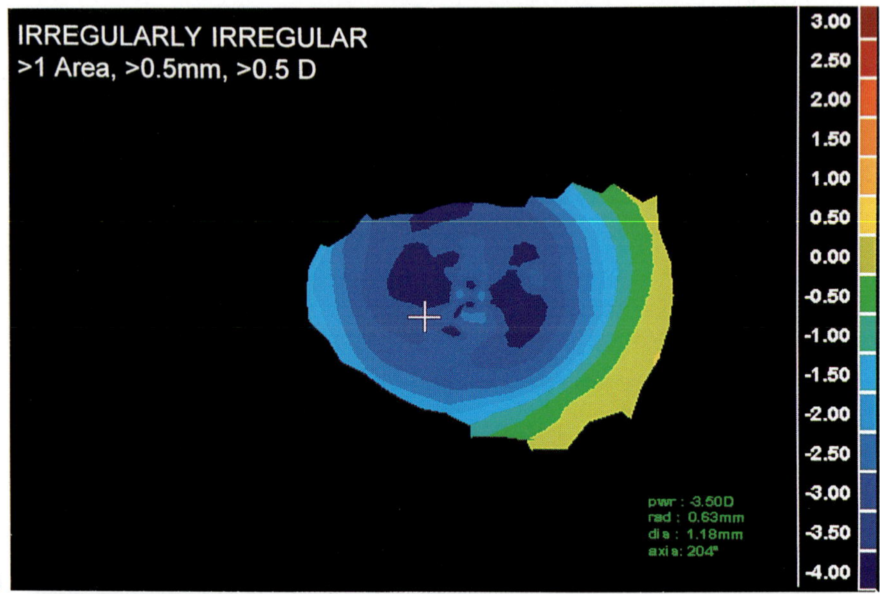

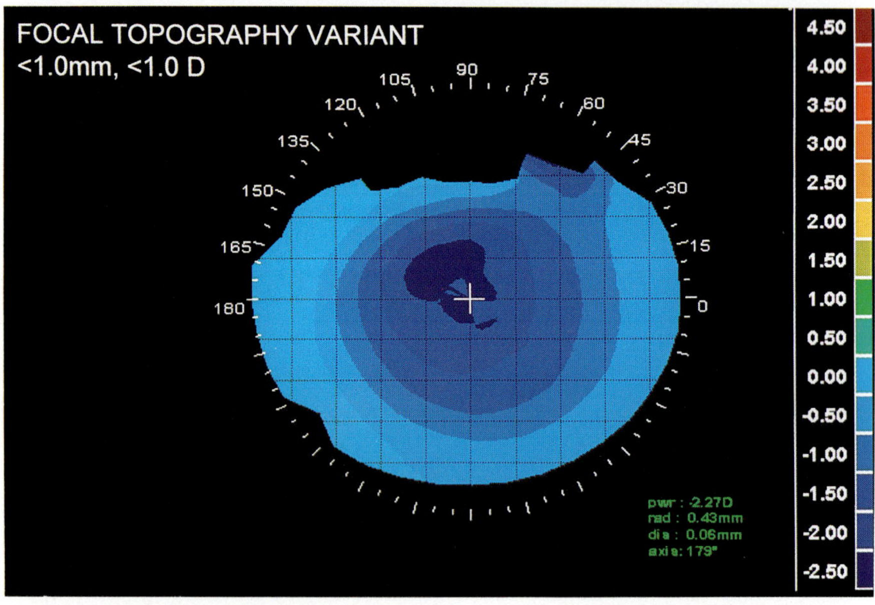

Figure 7-3. *Continued*   **(G)** Irregularly irregular. **(H)** Focal topography variant.

(Fig. 7-4). This is analogous to the treatment of a corneal nodule compared to treatment of a deeper stromal corneal scar—the corneal surface will be smoothed in the former and made more irregular in the latter. Topography instruments designed to measure surface elevation and contour characteristics may be useful in this assessment.[42] In addition, assessment of rigid contact lens fitting may aid in differentiating areas of corneal elevation from depressed areas of the corneal surface (Fig. 7-5).

As for other PTK procedures, care should be taken to minimize treatment to avoid postoperative overcorrections.

CASE 32

History and preoperative evaluation. A 36-year-old woman with a refractive error of -4.00–0.50 $\times$ 5 underwent uncomplicated excimer laser PRK to her right eye with an attempted correction of 3.9 diopters. She had previously undergone successful PRK to the left eye with postoperative uncorrected visual acuity of 20/20.

One month postoperatively, uncorrected visual acuity was 20/25 and refraction of plano-0.75 $\times$ 180 gave visual acuity of 20/20. However, the pa-

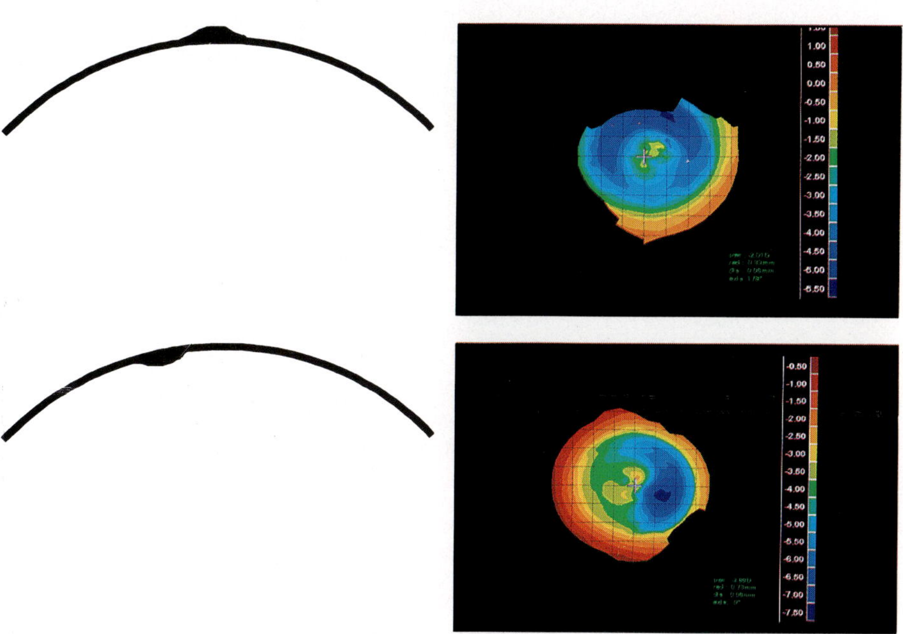

Figure 7-4.   **(Upper left)** Schematic of elevated central island. Excimer laser PTK to smooth this area would improve topography. **(Upper right)** Corresponding corneal topography map showing a central island. **(Lower left)** Schematic of depressed, but steep topography irregularity. PTK would worsen the topography. **(Lower right)** Corresponding corneal topography map showing a keyhole pattern.

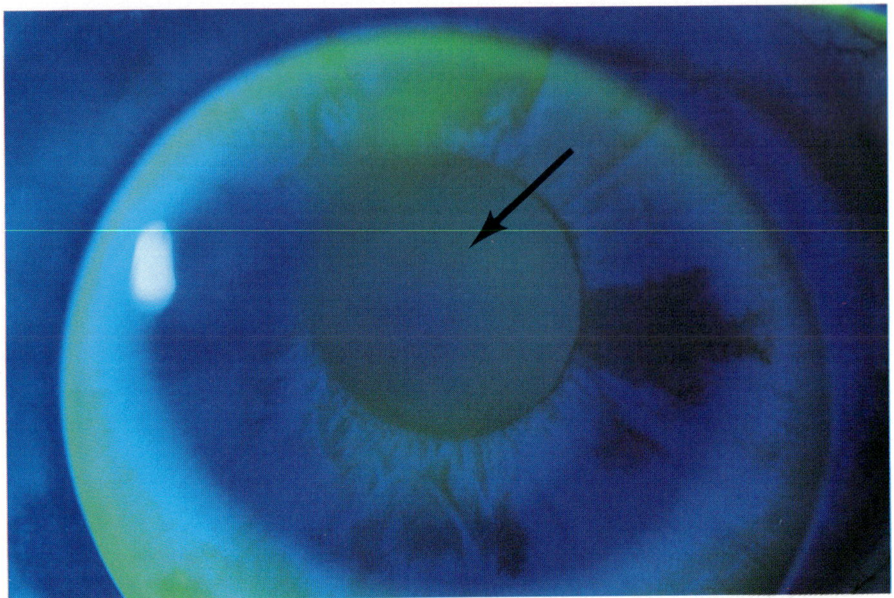

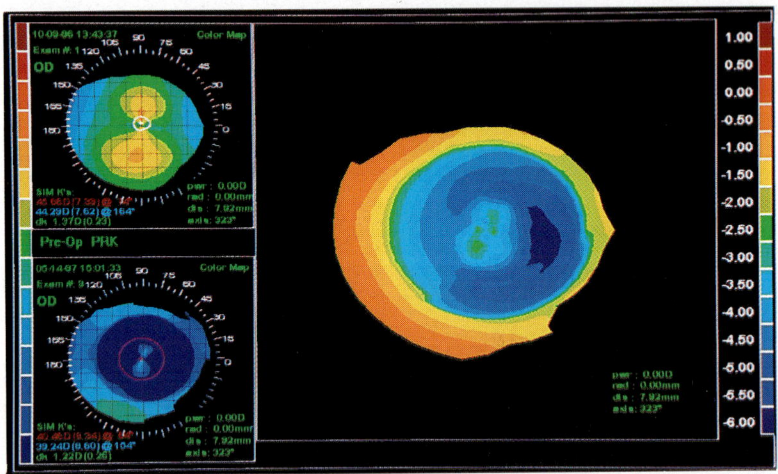

Figure 7-5.   **(A)** Demonstration of an elevated central island with a rigid contact lens. Note area of central lens touch by the central island (arrow) (photo courtesy of Donald Hersh, O.D.). **(B)** Corresponding videokeratography map showing the central island. **(Upper left)** Preoperative map. **(Lower left)** Postoperative map. **(Right)** Differential map.

tient complained of blurred vision with halos and monocular diplopia. A central island was noted on corneal topography analysis (Fig. 7-6A). Six months postoperatively, the patient's complaints persisted although uncorrected visual acuity was 20/25. Refraction remained plano-0.75 × 180 giving 20/20 visual acuity, although without amelioration of patient complaints. Rigid contact lens refraction did relieve the halo and diplopia symptoms.

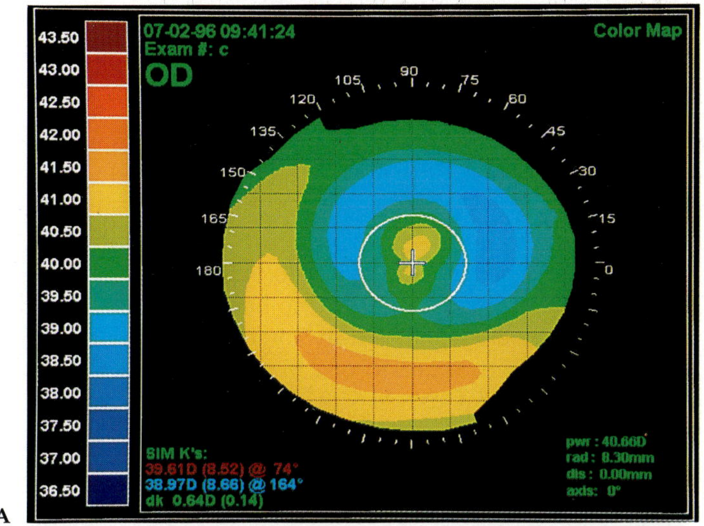

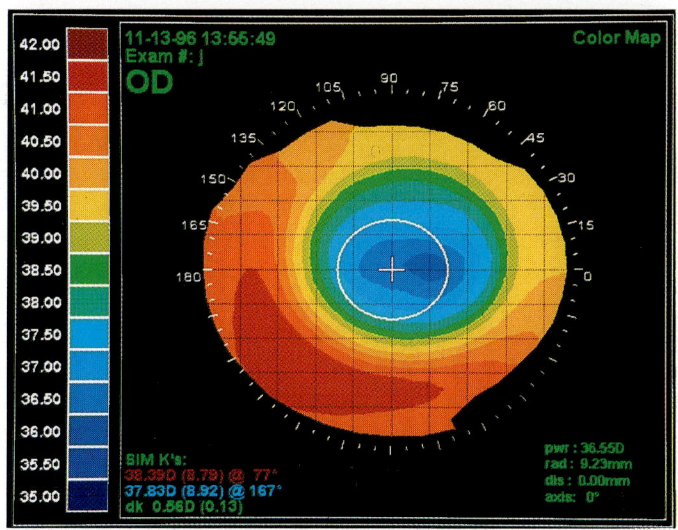

Figure 7-6. Case 32. **(A)** Following PRK (attempted correction 3.9D), uncorrected visual acuity is 20/25 and spectacle-corrected visual acuity is 20/20. The patient complained of poor vision, and a central island was found on corneal topography analysis. The island measured approximately 2 mm in diameter and 2 diopters in height. **(B)** One month following a 10 pulse, 2.0 mm PTK, the central island had been corrected and the patient's complaints of halo and diplopia had diminished.

Corneal topography mapping showed persistence of the central island. Since the patient did not want contact lens correction, the central island was assessed for retreatment.

Surgical therapy and outcome. The width and depth of the central island was calculated using the standard equation for sagittal depth of a spherical lens, $t = s^2 \times D/3$, where t = center thickness in microns, s = diameter of the lens, and D = power of the lens.[43,44] The approximate width of the island was 2 mm, and the dioptric height was approximately 2D. Thus, the sagittal height of the central island was calculated to be 2.67 microns ($2^2 \times 2/3$).

Epithelium was removed mechanically over a central 3 mm. Given the calculated depth of the central island of 2.67 microns and the expected ablation rate of corneal stromal tissue of 0.25 microns per pulse, a 10-pulse treatment using a 2.0-mm beam diameter was performed, being careful to keep the ablation centered.

One month postoperatively, the central island had been corrected (Fig. 7-6B), and the patient's complaints of halo and diplopia had diminished. However, uncorrected visual acuity had decreased to 20/25, and refraction had demonstrated a hyperopic shift to +1.75–0.50 × 15, giving 20/20 visual acuity.

Discussion. This case illustrates the importance of being conservative in retreatments after excimer laser PRK. Although this patient was happy with the diminution of her subjective optical symptomatology, refractive shifts may disturb an otherwise beneficial postoperative result. As for other corneal disorders, refractive considerations following excimer laser refractive surgery will, in part, dictate the advisability of treatment as well as the surgical strategy to be employed. Given these patients' expectations of refractive correction, such considerations may be of even greater importance in repeat excimer laser treatment of the PRK patient than in the PTK patient suffering previous corneal disease.

A similar approach can be used with other irregular topography patterns such as the keyhole and semicircular patterns. Relative elevation can be calculated using Munnerlyn's formula[43] as a starting point. The transepithelial approach is usually preferred since the epithelium over the elevated area may be thinner than over depressed areas. Thus, breakthrough to the stroma will often occur over the steeper, elevated area first, allowing PTK smoothing of this area while the remaining epithelium masks flat areas. However, epithelial removal must be carefully monitored and methycellulose placed over those exposed areas of stroma where ablation should be avoided.

In addition, some cases of PRK decentration can be treated with PTK.[44–49] A transepithelial approach again is used. The ablation is centered directly over the pupil or decentered an equivalent distance 180 degrees away from the original optical zone. Again, the epithelium frequently will be thinner at the edge of the previous optical zone, thus allowing smoothing of the edge and expansion and recentration of the ablation zone. Extreme care should be taken to avoid removing too much stromal tissue with consequent overcorrection.

Conclusions

As seen throughout this book, excimer laser phototherapeutic keratectomy has diverse applications in the treatment of corneal disorders as well as the amelioration of complications of refractive laser procedures. However, judicious patient selection and careful surgical planning are essential. When properly planned and executed, superficial corneal surgery with the excimer laser will be rewarded with a clear and optically functional postoperative cornea. The excimer laser thus represents a unique and important new tool to the corneal surgeon.

References

1. Waring GO, O'Connell MA, Maloney RK, Hagen KR, Brint SF, Durrie DS, Gordon M, Steinert RF. Photorefractive keratectomy for myopia using a 4.5-millimeter ablation zone. J Refract Surg 1995;11:170–180.
2. Salz JJ, Maguen E, Meburn AB, et al. A two-year experience with excimer laser photorefraction keratectomy with myopia. Ophthalmology 1993;100:873–882.
3. Weinstock S. Excimer laser keratectomy: One-year results with 100 myopic patients. CLAO Journal 1993;19:178–182.
4. Piebenga L, Matta C, Deitz M, Tauber J, Irvine JW, Sabates FN. Excimer photorefractive keratectomy for myopia. Ophthalmology 1993;100:1335–1345.
5. Orssaud C, Ganem S, Binaghi M, Patarin D, Putterman M. Photorefractive keratectomy in 176 eyes: one-year follow-up. Journal of Refractive and Corneal Surgery 1994;10:S199–S205.
6. Seiler T, Wollensack J. Myopic photorefractive keratectomy (PRK) with the excimer laser (193 nm): One-year follow-up. Ophthalmology 1991;98:1156–1163.
7. Maguen E, Salz JJ, Nesburn AB et al. Results of excimer laser photorefractive keratectomy for the correction of myopia. Ophthalmology 1994;101:1548–1556.
8. Talley AR, Hardten DR, Sher NA et al. Results one year after using the 193-nm excimer laser for photorefractive keratectomy in mild to moderate myopia. Am J Ophthalmol 1994;118:304–311.
9. Sher NA, Hardten DR, Fundingsland B. 193-nm excimer photorefractive keratectomy in high myopia. Ophthalmology 1994;101:1575–1582.
10. Epstein D, Fagerholm P, Hamberg NH, Tengroth B. Twenty-four-month follow-up of excimer laser photorefractive keratectomy for myopia. Refractive and visual acuity results. Ophthalmology 1994;101(9):1558–1563.
11. Gartry DS, Kerr Muir MG, Marshall J. Excimer laser photorefractive keratectomy. Ophthalmology 1992;99:1209–1219.
12. Shah SI, Hersh PS. Clinical outcomes of photorefractive keratectomy for myopia using a 6.0 mm beam diameter. J Refract Surg 1996;12:341–351.
13. Hersh PS, Stulting D, Steinert RF, Waring GO, Thompson K, Doney K, O'Connell M. Results of phase III photoreactive keratectomy for myopia. Ophthalmology 1997;104.
14. Tuft S, Marshall J, Rothery S. Stromal remodeling following photorefractive keratectomy. Lasers in Ophthalmology 1981;1:77–183.
15. Tuft SJ, Zabel RW, Marshall J. Corneal repair following keratectomy: A comparison between conventional surgery and laser photoablation. Invest Ophthalmol Vis Sci 1989;30:1769–1777.

16. Braunstein RE, Jain S, McCally RL, Stark WJ, Connolly PJ, Azar D. Objective measurement of corneal light scattering after excimer laser keratectomy. Ophthalmology 1996;103:439–443.

17. Durrie D, Lesher W, Cavanaugh TB. Classification of variable clinical response after photorefractive keratectomy for myopia. J. Refract Surg 1995;11:341–347.

18. Carr J, Patel R, Hersh PS. Management of late corneal haze following photorefractive keratectomy. J Refractive Surg 1995;11(suppl):309–313.

19. Seiler T, Derse M, Pham T. Repeated excimer laser treatment after photorefractive keratectomy. Arch Ophthalmol 1992;110:1230–1233.

20. Epstein D, Tengroth B, Fagerholm P, Hamberg NH. Excimer retreatment of regression after photorefractive keratectomy. Am J Ophthalmol 1994;117(4):456–461.

21. Hersh PS, Schwartz-Goldstein BH, Summit PRK Topography Study Group. Corneal Topography of Phase III excimer laser photorefractive keratectomy: Characterization and clinical effects of treatment zone topography. Ophthalmology 1995;102:963–978.

22. Hersh PS, Shah S, Geiger D, Holladay J, Summit Photorefractive Keratectomy Topography Study Group. Corneal optical irregularity after excimer laser photorefractive keratectomy. J Cat Refract Surg 1996;22:197–204.

23. Hersh PS, Shah SI, Summit Photorefractive Keratectomy Topography Study Group. Corneal topography of excimer laser photorefractive keratectomy using a 6.0 mm beam diameter. Ophthalmology (in press).

24. Verdon W, Bullimore M, Maloney RK. Visual performance after photorefractive keratectomy. Arch Ophthalmol 1996;114:1465–1472.

25. Klyce SD, Smolek MK. Corneal topography of excimer laser photorefractive keratectomy. J Cataract Refract Surg 1993;19(suppl):122–129.

26. Colin J, Cochener B, Gallinaro C. Central steep islands immediately following excimer photorefractive keratectomy for myopia (letter). J Refract Corneal Surg 1993;9:395–396.

27. Hersh PS, Shah S, Holladay JT. Corneal asphericity following excimer laser photorefractive keratectomy. Ophth Surg Lasers 1996;27S:421–428.

28. Lin DTC, Sutton HF, Berman M. Corneal topography following excimer photorefractive keratectomy for myopia. J Cataract Refract Surg 1993;19:149–154.

29. Hersh PS, Shah S, Summit PRK Topography Study Group. Corneal topography of 6.0 mm excimer laser photorefractive keratectomy. Ophthalmology 1997;104:1333–1342.

30. Wilson SE, Klyce SD, McDonald MB et al. Changes in corneal topography after excimer laser photorefractive keratectomy for myopia. Ophthalmology 1991;98:1338–1347.

31. Maguire L, Bechara S. Epithelial distortions at the ablation zone margin after excimer laser photorefractive keratectomy for myopia. Am J Ophthalmol 1991;117:809–810.

32. Hersh PS, Shah S, Geiger D, Holladay J. Corneal optical irregularity after excimer laser photorefractive keratectomy. J Cat Refract Surg 1996;22:197–204.

33. Hersh PS, Shah SI, Durrie D. Diplopia following excimer laser photorefractive keratectomy. Ophth Surg Lasers 1996;27:315–317.

34. Meyer JC, Stulting RD, Thompson KP, Durrie D. Late onset corneal scar after excimer laser photorefractive keratectomy. Am J Ophthalmol 1996;121:529–539.

35. Grimm B, Waring GO, Ibrahim O. Regional variation in corneal topography and wound healing following photorefractive keratectomy. J Refract Surg 1995;11:348–357.

36. Hersh P, Ophthalmic Surgical Procedures. Boston: Little, Brown; 1988:221–224.

37. Loewenstein A, Lipshitz I, Lazar M. Scraping of epithelium for treatment of undercorrection and haze after photorefractive keratectomy. J Refract Corneal Surg 1994;10:S274–S276.

38. Fitzsimmons TD, Fagerholm P, Tengroth B. Steroid treatment of myopic regression: Acute refractive and topographic changes in excimer photorefractive keratectomy patients. Cornea 1993;12(4):358–361.

39. Gartry D, Kerr Muir M, Lohmann CP, Marshall J. The effect of topical corticosteroids on refractive outcome and corneal haze after photorefractive keratectomy: A prospective, randomized, double-blind trial. Arch Ophthalmol 1992;110:944–952.

40. O'Brart DP, Lohmann CP, Klonos G et al. The effects of topical corticosteroids and plasmin inhibitors on refractive outcome, haze, and visual performance after photorefractive keratectomy: A prospective, randomized, observer-masked study. Ophthalmology 1994;101(9): 1565–1574.

41. Fitzsimmons TD, Fagerholm P, Tengroth B. Steroid treatment of myopic regression: Acute refractive and topographic changes in excimer photorefractive keratectomy patients. Cornea 1993;12:358–361.

42. Belin MW, Litoff D, Strobs JT, Winn SS, Smith RS. The PAR Technology corneal topography system. J Refractive Corneal Surgery 1993;8:88–96.
43. Munnerlyn CR, Koons SJ, Marshall J. Photorefractive keratectomy: A technique for laser refractive surgery. J Cataract Refract Surg 1988;14:46–52.
44. Blaker JW, Hersh PS. Theoretical and clinical effect of corneal curvature on excimer laser photorefractive keratectomy. Refractive Corneal Surg 1994;10:571–574.
45. O'Brart DP, Gartry DS, Lohmann CP, Muir MG, Marshall J. Excimer laser photorefractive keratectomy for myopia: Comparison of 4.00 and 5.00 millimeter ablation zones. J Refract Corneal Surg 1994;10:87–94.
46. O'Brart DPS, Corbett MC, Lohmann CP, Kerr Muir MG, Marshall J. The effects of ablation diameter on the outcome of excimer laser photorefractive keratectomy: A prospective, randomized, double-blind study. Arch Ophthalmol 1995;113:438–443.
47. Uozato H, Guyton DL. Centering corneal surgical procedures. Am J Ophthalmol 1987;103:264–275.
48. Schwartz-Goldstein BH, Hersh PS, Summit PRK Topography Study Group. Corneal topography of Phase III excimer laser photorefractive keratectomy: Optical zone centration analysis. Ophthalmology 1995;102:951–962.
49. Maloney RK. Corneal topography and optical zone location in photorefractive keratectomy. J Refract Corneal Surg 1990;6:363–371.
50. Hersh PS, Rice BA, Baer JC, Wells PA, Lynch SE, McGuigan LJB, Foster CS. Topical nonsteroidal agents and corneal wound healing. Arch Ophthalmol 1990;108:577–583.

Addendum: Case Studies

Case 1 (Figs. 3–3, 3–4). Manual superficial keratectomy for excision of paracentral nodule.

Case 2 (Figs. 3–5 to 3–7). Manual superficial keratectomy of subepithelial fibrous plaque.

Case 3 (Fig. 3–11). PTK treatment of irregular astigmatism.

Case 4 (Fig. 3–13). General large area PTK using the polishing technique and masking methylcellulose to treat Reis-Buckler's dystrophy.

Case 5 (Fig. 3–14). General large area PTK using the polishing technique and masking methylcellulose to treat lattice corneal dystrophy.

Case 6 (Fig. 3–17). Combined manual superficial keratectomy and PTK to treat calcific band keratopathy.

Case 7 (Fig. 3–19). Combined manual superficial keratectomy and PTK to treat calcific band keratopathy secondary to juvenille rheumatoid arthritis.

Case 8 (Fig. 3–21). Focal PTK to treat plaquelike, fibrous scar secondary to trauma.

Case 9 (Fig. 3–22). Focal PTK to treat Salzmann's nodule.

Case 10 (Fig. 3–23). Focal PTK to treat elevated nodule.

Case 11 (Fig. 3–25). Removal of a superficial scar, secondary to herpes keratitis, by technique 1—general PTK polishing technique.

Case 12 (Fig. 3–27). Removal of a central corneal scar by technique 2—wide beam diameter directly ablates scar, with a peripheral annulus of treatment.

Case 13 (Fig. 3–30). PTK treatment of recurrent epithelial erosion.

Case 14 (Fig. 4–5). Treatment of smooth climatic droplet keratopathy.

Case 15 (Fig. 4–6). Treatment of irregular climatic droplet keratopathy.

Case 16 (Fig. 5–3). Recurrence of an optically poor epithelial surface following PTK.

Case 17 (Fig. 5–4). Microbial keratitis following PTK for climatic droplet keratopathy.

Case 18 (Fig. 5–5). Microbial keratitis following PTK for climatic droplet keratopathy.

Case 19 (Fig. 5–6). Corneal graft rejection following PTK for treatment of recurrent lattice dystrophy.

Case 20 (Fig. 5–7). Recurrence of herpes simplex dendritic keratitis following PTK for anterior stromal scarring.

Case 21 (Fig. 5–8). Recurrence of Reis-Bucklers' corneal dystrophy following manual superficial keratectomy and again following PTK.

154

Case 22 (Fig. 6–2). Improvement in corneal topography following PTK for Saltzmann's nodular degeneration.

Case 23 (Fig. 6–3). Improvement in corneal topography following combined focal manual keratectomy and PTK for a fibrous scar.

Case 24 (Fig. 6–4). Improvement in corneal topography following general large area PTK.

Case 25 (Fig. 6–1). Change in corneal topography showing increased irregularity following PTK for a herpetic stromal scar.

Case 26 (Fig. 6–5). Hyperopic shift following large area general PTK for Reis-Buckler's dystrophy.

Case 27 (Fig. 6–8). Midperipheral annulus of treatment to minimize hyperopic shift in Reis-Buckler's patient.

Case 28 (Fig. 6–9). Midperipheral annulus of treatment to minimize hyperopic shift in a patient with a superficial corneal scar.

Case 29 (Fig. 6–10). Focal treatment of steep areas of the cornea to decrease irregular astigmatism.

Case 30 (Fig. 7–1). Ring scar following PRK treated with PTK.

Case 31 (Fig. 7–2). Fibrous corneal scar following PRK treated first with mechanical superficial keratectomy and then with PTK.

Case 32 Fig. 7–6). Treatment of central island following PRK.

Index

Ablation rate, 5–6, 117
Ablative photodecomposition, 2–4
Acyclovir, use in herpetic keratitis, 73
Amyloid degeneration, 37
Anterior stromal pathology, 21–23, 25, 30, 32
Antibiotics, postoperatively, 73
Antiviral agents, use in herpetic keratitis, 73, 101
Apical nodules in keratoconus, 37, 60
Apical scarring of keratoconus, 3, 17, 19, 20
Astigmatism
   clinical results, 79, 80
   irregular, 29, 32, 33, 37, 43, 45, 48, 50, 51, 127

Bandage soft contact lens, 90, 91, 94
Band keratopathy, 13, 15, 18, 22, 26–28, 31, 32, 38
   clinical results, 75, 76, 81
   combined manual superficial keratectomy and PTK and, 37, 56–60
Beam diameters, 5, 7
Beam homogenization, 5
Beam profile, 5–7
Bowman's pathology, 21–24, 29–32

Calcific band keratopathy, 37, 38, 56–60, 81
Carcinogenesis, 8
Case selection, 2, 11–33
   clinical presentation and, 14

factors in, 11
primary diagnosis and, 14
surgical decision making. *See* Surgical decision making
Central island corneal topography, 142, 145, 147–150
Climatic droplet keratopathy, 13, 15, 16, 18, 22–26, 37
   clinical results, 81–86
   complications associated with surgery, 91, 94–97
Clinical presentation, 14
Clinical results, 75–87
   See also Complications
Collagen gels, 46
Complications, 2, 89–128
   corneal graft reaction, 95, 97, 99, 100
   corneal infection, 94–98
   epithelialization problems, 89–94
   of photorefractive keratectomy (PRK). *See* Photorefractive keratectomy (PRK) complications, PTK for
   recurrence of disease, 101–103
   recurrent herpes simplex keratitis, 99, 101
   refractive shifts. *See* Refractive shifts
   stromal haze and scarring, 95
   subsequent penetrating keratoplasty, 102
   topographic. *See* Corneal topographic changes
Contact lenses, bandage, 90, 91, 94

Contact lens keratopathy, 37, 76,
91–93
Contrast sensitivity, decreased, 129,
130
Corneal degenerations, 37
See also names of specific degenerations
Corneal dystrophies, 37, 44, 75, 81,
101
See also names of specific dystrophies
Corneal flattening following PTK,
117–119
Corneal graft reaction, 95, 97, 99, 100
Corneal haze following photorefractive keratectomy
as indication for PTK, 129
treatment, 130–141
Corneal infection, 94–98
Corneal irregularities, 37, 44, 48
See also names of specific irregularities
Corneal opacities, 29, 44, 60, 95
See also Corneal haze following
photorefractive keratectomy
Corneal scar removal. *See* Superficial scar removal
Corneal scarring following photorefractive keratectomy
as indication for PTK, 129
treatment, 130–141
Corneal steepening, 118, 119
Corneal topographic abnormalities
following photorefractive keratectomy
as indication for PTK, 129
treatment, 141–150
Corneal topographic changes:
cases, 105–113
minimization of, 119–126
treatment, 127
types
central island, 142, 145, 147–
150

focal topography variant, 142,
146
homogeneous, 142, 143
keyhole, 142, 145, 150
semicircular, 142, 144, 150
Corticosteroids, 73, 90, 95, 99, 101,
135

Diclofenac, 133, 141
Diplopia, monocular, 129–131, 142,
148
Disease, recurrence of, 101–103

Effluent plume, 4, 7
Energy meter, 6
Energy profiles, 5, 6
Epithelial adherence disorders, 29,
37
contact lens keratopathy, 37, 76,
91–93
See also Epithelial basement membrane dystrophy
Epithelial basement membrane dystrophy, 13, 15, 16, 18, 22–24, 31,
37
clinical results, 75–78
recurrence of, 101
recurrent epithelial erosion syndrome and, 70–73, 75, 76, 113,
114
Epithelial fluorescence, 47
Epithelialization problems, 89–94
Excimer, defined, 2
Excimer laser surgery. *See* Phototherapeutic keratectomy (PTK)

Fluence, 4
Fluorine, 2, 3
Fluoromethalone, 73, 133, 141
Fluroquinolone, 94
Focal irregularities following surgery or infection, 37
Focal nodules, 37, 60
Focal smoothing, 37, 60–66, 76, 113,
114

Focal topography variant, 142, 146
Functional objectives, 23, 26, 29–31

General large area PTK, 37, 44–56,
    76, 113, 114
Glare, 129, 130, 133–135, 142
Granular dystrophy, 13, 15, 18, 19,
    21, 22, 37

Halo, 129, 133–135, 142, 148
Herpes simplex keratitis, 73, 99, 101
Herpetic keratitis scars, 37, 106,
    112–113
Homogeneous corneal topography,
    142, 143
Hyperopic PTK technique, 68–70,
    120–126

Immunological corneal graft reac-
    tion, 95, 97, 99, 100
Infection:
    corneal, 94–98
    focal irregularities following, 37
Irregular astigmatism, 29, 32, 33, 37,
    43, 45, 48, 50, 51, 127
Irregular corneal surface, 29
Irregularly irregular corneal topog-
    raphy, 142, 146

Keratectomy. *See* Manual superficial
    keratectomy; Phototherapeutic
    keratectomy (PTK)
Keratitis
    herpes simplex, 73, 99, 101
    microbial, 94–98
Keratoconus
    apical nodules in, 37, 60
    laser treatment of raised nodular
        scars in patients with, 85
Keyhole corneal topography, 142,
    145, 150

Laser-assisted superficial keratec-
    tomy. *See* Phototherapeutic ker-
    atectomy (PTK)

Lattice dystrophy, 13, 15, 18, 22
    clinical results, 76
    recurrent, corneal grafts and, 95,
        97, 99
    surgical techniques for, 37, 44, 53,
        55, 56
Lensometer, 6
Limbal stem cell population, 89
Lubrication, 73, 90

Macular corneal dystrophy, 22–23,
    25
Manual superficial keratectomy:
    combined with PTK, 37, 56–60,
        113, 114
    vs. PTK, 12–13
    technique, 38–46
Meesman's dystrophy, 15, 18, 37
Methylcellulose, 37, 45–47, 48, 53,
    66, 68, 69, 117
Microbial keratitis, 94–98
Mutagenesis, 8

Nodular pathology, 17, 19, 20, 26,
    29–30

Optical zone, 15, 26, 29–32

Paracentral zone, 15–16, 26, 30, 32
Patient complaints, 11
Pattern assessment, 17–21, 26
Penetrating keratoplasty, subse-
    quent, 102
Peripheral zone, 16, 18, 26, 30, 33
Persistent epithelial defects, 13
Photorefractive keratectomy (PRK)
    complications, PTK for, 129–
    151
    indications, 129
    treatment of corneal haze and
        scars, 130–141
    treatment of corneal topography
        irregularities, 141–150

Phototherapeutic keratectomy
(PTK)
  case selection. *See* Case selection
  clinical results, 75–87
  combined with manual superfi-
    cial keratectomy, 37, 56–60, 78,
    113, 114
  complications. *See* Complications
    for complications of photore-
    fractive keratectomy (PRK),
    Photorefractive keratectomy
    (PRK) complications, PTK for
  focal smoothing, 37, 60–66, 78,
    113, 114
  general large area, 37, 44–56, 113,
    114
  vs. manual superficial keratec-
    tomy, 12–13
  postoperative management, 73
  preoperative preparation, 36–37
  recurrent epithelial membrane
    syndrome, 70–73, 113, 114
  superficial scar removal, 37, 66–
    70, 113, 114
  technology. *See* Technology
Pilocarpine, 37
Postinfectious scarring, 15–20, 22,
  81
Post-pterygium scarring, 15
Post-traumatic corneal epithelial
  erosions, 16
Pre-Bowman's pathology, 21–24,
  30–31
Preoperative laser calibration, 5–6
Pterygium, 16, 18–20, 33, 37
PTK. *See* Phototherapeutic keratectomy (PTK)

Recurrence of disease, 101–103
Recurrent corneal intraepithelial
  dysplasia, 85, 87
Recurrent dystrophies, 15
Recurrent epithelial erosion syn-
  drome, 70–73, 76, 85, 95
Recurrent herpes simplex keratitis,
  99, 101

Re-epithelialization, 8, 82, 84, 90–94
Refractive accuracy, 6
Refractive shifts:
  case, 115–117
  mechanism of, 117–119
  minimization of, 119–126
  treatment of, 127
  by treatment strategy, 113, 114
Reis-Buckler's dystrophy, 13–15, 18,
  19, 21, 22, 23, 26, 31
  recurrence of, 102, 103
  refractive shifts and, 115–117,
    123–125
  surgical techniques for, 37, 44, 46,
    50, 52–53

Salzmann's nodular degeneration,
  13, 17, 37
  clinical results, 75, 76, 81
  complications, 91, 101, 105–106,
    108–109
  focal smoothing and, 60, 62–63
Salzmann's nodules, 16, 32, 40, 120
Scars
  corneal, following photorefractive
    keratectomy. *See* Corneal scar-
    ring following photorefractive
    keratectomy
  herpetic keratitis, 37, 106, 112–
    113
  of keratoconus, apical. *See* Proud
    nebulae
  postinfectious, 15–20, 22, 81
  post-pterygium, 15
  raised nodular, in patients with
    keratoconus, 85
  stromal, 95, 120
  superficial, removal of. *See* Super-
    ficial scar removal
Schneider's crystalline dystrophy,
  37
Segmental pathology, 17–20, 26,
  29–30
Semicircular corneal topography,
  142, 144, 150
Side effects. *See* Complications

Slit lamp, 48, 49
Staphylococcus, 94, 96
Streptococcus pneumonia 94, 98
Stromal haze, 95
Stromal pathology, 21–23, 25, 30, 32
Stromal scars, 95, 120
Superficial scar removal, 13, 37
    clinical results, 75–78, 81
    refractive shifts and, 68, 70, 113,
        114, 120–126
    technique, 66–70
Surgery, complications associated
        with. *See* Complications
Surgical decision making
    manual superficial keratectomy
        vs. PTK, 12–13
    therapeutic algorithm, 26, 29–33
    therapeutic parameters, 14–26
Surgical strategies, 2, 36–73
    combined manual superficial ker-
        atectomy and PTK, 37, 56–60,
        113, 114
    epithilial basement membrane
        dystrophy, 13, 15, 16, 18, 22–24,
        31, 37
    focal smoothing, 37, 60–66, 76,
        113, 114
    general large-area PTK, 37, 44–
        56, 76, 113, 114
    manual superficial keratectomy,
        38–46
    postoperative management, 73
    preoperative preparation, 36–37
    PTK. *See* Phototherapeutic kera-
        tectomy (PTK)
    recurrent epithilial erosion syn-
        drome, 70–73, 76, 85, 95

    superficial scar removal, 66–70
Surgical trauma, minimization of,
    1–2

Tarsorrhapy, 90
Technology, 1–9
    delivery, 5–7
    laser-tissue interaction, 7
    principles, 2–5
    wound healing, 7–9
Tetracycline derivatives, 90
Therapeutic algorithm, 26, 29–33
Therapeutic parameters, 14–26
Thermal damage, 7
Tissue-laser interaction, 7
Tissue removal, minimization of,
    1–2
Topographic abnormalities. *See* Cor-
    neal topographic abnormalities
    following photorefractive kera-
    tectomy
Topographic changes. *See* Corneal
    topographic changes
Toric-against-axis corneal topogra-
    phy, 142, 144
Toric-with-axis corneal topography,
    142, 143
Traumatic scars, 37

U.S. Food and Drug Administration
    (FDA), 1

Vertical assessment, 18, 22–25
Visual acuity, clinical results, 75–87
Visual objectives, 23

Wavelength, 2, 3
Wound healing, 7–9